Women and the AIDS Crisis

Diane Richardson

London

First published in 1987 by
Pandora Press
(Routledge & Kegan Paul Ltd)
11 New Fetter Lane, London EC4P 4EE

Set in Palatino, 10 on 12pt.
by Columns of Reading
and printed in the British Isles
by the Guernsey Press Co. Ltd
Guernsey, Channel Islands

British Library Cataloguing in Publication data

Richardson, Diane
Women and the AIDS crisis.
1. AIDS (Disease)
I. Title
616.9'792   RC607.A26

ISBN 0-86358-209-5 (c)
      0-86358-189-7 (pb)

Contents

Acknowledgments   ix
Introduction   1

1 What is AIDS?   3
What causes AIDS?   6
Where did AIDS originate?   8
How serious is AIDS?   10
How is AIDS transmitted?   12
Who gets AIDS?   17
What are the symptoms of AIDS?   19
Can AIDS be treated?   20

2 AIDS in women   24
High-risk groups   24
Injecting drug users   26
Sexual transmission   30
Sexual partners of men at risk   33
Prostitutes   35
Rape   39
African women   40
Haitian women   44
Blood transfusions   45
Pregnancy   47
Artificial insemination   51

3   Lesbians and AIDS   55
Who is at risk?   57
Safer sex   61
Lesbians with AIDS   66

4   Safer sex   68
How can a woman reduce her risk of AIDS?   70
Anal sex   73
Vaginal intercourse   76
Oral sex   78
Kissing   79
Masturbation   80
Safe sex   80

5   Living with AIDS   82
Finding out   82
AIDS discrimination   86
Isolation   86
Anxiety   88
Depression   91
Sexuality   95

6   Caring for people with AIDS   97
The experience of care   98
A labour of love   99
Caring means work   104
Women doing AIDS work   106
Carers of children with AIDS   109

7   Policies and prevention   114
Education   115
Health and social services   119
Housing   123
AIDS discrimination – the antibody test   125

8   The challenge of AIDS   129

Afterword 132

Note on sources 135

Resources list 137

Glossary 142

Index 146

Acknowledgments

When Philippa Brewster, my editor, first suggested I write a book on women and AIDS I was reluctant. Now, having finished it, I am grateful to her for asking me. I also want to thank her for her support and editorial work. Linda Semple was also a great help in editing the book. She gave me constructive criticism which has helped to improve the quality of the book. I also want to thank Liz Young at Pandora, who was tireless in her efforts to find answers to difficult questions. My additional thanks to Lisa Power of the Angel Project. Thanks also to Val Squire, Margaret Jaram, Christine Bell, Sheila Fuller and Sylvia Parkin for typing the manuscript.

Various organisations concerned with AIDS were helpful in providing me with information and advice. I would like to thank them, in particular the Terrence Higgins Trust, the Haemophilia Society, the Shanti Project and Project Aware in San Francisco, the Gay Men's Health Crisis in New York, and the San Francisco AIDS Foundation. I would also like to thank Janet Green at the Terrence Higgins Trust and Fran Pierce at the Middlesex Hospital for their time and patience in answering my questions.

Most women who are infected with HIV, or are caring for someone who is, are reluctant to be interviewed. For this reason I owe a very special thanks to the women I spoke to who had the courage to share their experiences. Knowing their fears, I am most grateful to them.

Finally, I want to thank JW for cheering me up, and my friends Jackie Davis, Dorothy Dixon-Barrow, Mal Finch, Libby Hawkins, Ankie Hoogvelt and Ann Watkinson. As they know this has been, in many ways, a difficult book to write and their practical and emotional support has helped greatly in its completion.

Sheffield
November 1986

Introduction

The first cases of AIDS were reported in 1981, in the United States. Initially it seemed to be a disease which only affected gay men. Soon, however, it became clear that other groups of people – injecting drug users, haemophiliacs, Haitian immigrants – were catching it. This, and the discovery that AIDS could be spread through blood transfusion, which meant that *anyone* might conceivably get it, captured the media's attention. Stories about AIDS began to appear with great frequency, and by mid-1983 AIDS hysteria had set in.

Interestingly, despite the widespread attention AIDS has received from the media, and the evidence that it can be transmitted heterosexually, most people don't really expect AIDS to affect them. If they think about it at all it is as 'the gay plague', a disease that happens to 'other' people. This is especially likely to be true of women. Yet women certainly do get AIDS. In Africa the disease is believed to have affected thousands of women, while in Europe and America, although the majority of people with AIDS are gay or bisexual men, a significant number of women have the disease. Most of them are women who inject drugs, some are sexual partners of drug users, haemophiliacs, or bisexual men, and a smaller number are recipients of infected blood transfusions.

As AIDS becomes more widespread women who may

once have seen the disease as largely confined to men are becoming more concerned about their own risks of infection. This book is aimed at them, as well as the women who already have AIDS or the virus which causes it. It is also for women who care for people with AIDS. It provides what is currently lacking: a clear and informative account of the issues which AIDS raises for women. In addition to providing important information, the book also challenges the racism, sexism and homophobia surrounding the disease.

There is so much that we still don't know or understand about AIDS that to write about it at the moment is very difficult. New discoveries are being made all the time and, consequently, some of the information in this book may need to be changed in the light of those. AIDS is also difficult to write about for other reasons. It is a tragic illness. Disfiguring and debilitating to those who have it, AIDS primarily affects the young, and is ultimately fatal. Living in San Francisco for six months during 1985 I became acutely aware of how AIDS can affect both individuals and communities. What I remember, however, is not just the sadness and the anger but also the bravery and the struggle to survive.

AIDS is not a 'gay disease'; it affects those who are heterosexual as well as those who are gay, women as well as men. It is a social problem which we all need to be concerned about. At the same time panic and hysteria are not helpful. It is hoped that this book will help to remove many fears about AIDS, whilst providing women at risk with information about how to avoid getting it.

1 What is AIDS?

Acquired Immune Deficiency Syndrome or, as it is more commonly known, AIDS, is a new and fatal disease. It is caused by a virus called human immunodeficiency virus or HIV for short. The credit for discovery of this virus is shared between French and American researchers, although it was the team at the Pasteur Institute in Paris, led by Dr Luc Montagnier, who first announced its discovery early in 1983. The name they gave to the virus was LAV, or lymphadenopathy associated virus. The American team, led by Dr Robert Gallo, called the virus HTLV-3 or human T-cell lymphotropic virus type-3. To simplify matters researchers have now agreed to use the term HIV.

A virus is one of a group of extremely small micro-organisms that can only survive inside the cells of other living creatures. HIV attacks the body's immune system. When the immune system is impaired, the body becomes vulnerable to infections and cancers which healthy people with intact immune systems can ward off. These illnesses are sometimes referred to as 'opportunistic infections', because they take advantage of the opportunity offered by the body's weakened immunity to enter and do their damage. The most common illnesses found in people with AIDS are a rare form of pneumonia known as pneumocystis carinii pneumonia (PCP), and a rare form of skin cancer called Kaposi's sarcoma (KS). It is the cancers and the opportunistic infections, not AIDS itself, that cause death. This usually occurs within two or three years of being diagnosed as having AIDS. People with KS have a better chance of surviving than those with opportunistic infections. However, no one has yet been known to recover from AIDS.

HIV can cause a range of conditions, of which AIDS is the worst. For example, it can lead to persistent swelling of the lymph nodes. People in whom this is the only symptom of HIV infection are said to have persistent generalised lymphadenopathy or PGL. Other people may have more serious symptoms, but still not show any signs of the opportunistic infections and cancers that are associated with AIDS. The Americans have termed this AIDS-related complex or ARC. This is estimated to affect up to ten times as many people as are diagnosed as having AIDS. Though it is serious, AIDS-related complex is not necessarily fatal. A significant proportion of those with ARC do however go on to develop AIDS.

A much larger group, some estimate as many as a hundred times the number of people with AIDS, are infected with HIV yet show no symptoms. Whether someone has been infected with HIV can be determined by the HIV antibody test. This is a blood test which detects the presence or absence of antibodies to the virus. It indicates only whether a person has at some time been infected with HIV. It cannot determine whether a person has AIDS or will develop AIDS in the future. A positive test result means that antibodies to HIV are present, and that the virus has been in the body at some time and has caused the body to react to it. The test does not measure infectiousness, though at present it must be assumed that anyone who is antibody positive is probably capable of passing the virus on to someone else. A negative result to the test *usually* means that the virus is not present. However as the test sometimes produces false negatives, a negative test result does not necessarily mean that someone is free from infection. Also, it takes a few months after infection for the body to produce antibodies to HIV. This means that if someone were tested shortly after having been infected the test would be negative.

There are two aspects to the question of whether or not someone should take the test. Will knowing their test result make them more or less likely to infect others, and will it help their own physical and mental health?

If a person is extremely anxious about the possibility that they may have been infected with HIV it *may* be beneficial to have the test. Knowing that you are antibody positive also gives you a chance to alter your lifestyle in ways that may, possibly, reduce your risk of developing AIDS (see page 85). Many people, however, feel there is little point in taking the test because there is no effective treatment available for those who discover they are antibody positive, and because the advice offered is the same whether the test result is positive or negative.

Early studies suggested that about one in ten people infected with the virus went on to develop AIDS. It now seems that this figure was too low. More recent estimates are that between 20 and 30 per cent of those infected with HIV get AIDS. Others, as I have already described, may develop less serious illnesses.

Even if HIV does not affect a person's immune system, it may have other serious consequences. It seems HIV affects and damages the brain, causing a variety of psychological effects including memory loss, personality disturbance and dementia. No one knows as yet why the virus affects different people in such different ways.

It is not as yet possible to say what the long-term effects of HIV infection might be. No one knows how many more people who have the virus are likely to become ill in the future.

At the time of writing, between 30,000 and 40,000 people are thought to have been infected with HIV in the United Kingdom. It is vital that all those who know they are infected realise that, healthy or not, they could be infectious and should take precautions to avoid the possibility of transmitting the virus to others. Not to do so might mean someone else's death due to AIDS.

The difficulty with this is the long incubation period. It can take anything from a few months to several years after infection with HIV for symptoms to develop. Consequently, many people who are infected with the virus don't know they are.

The kinds of precautions you should take if you think that you may be infected are described later.

What causes AIDS?

The cause of AIDS is not yet fully understood. We know that the virus HIV must be present in the body for AIDS to occur. However the fact that not all of those infected with the virus go on to develop AIDS suggests that other factors are involved. Alcohol or drug use, poor nutrition, high stress levels, and frequent exposure to other diseases, especially sexually transmitted diseases, have all been suggested as possibilities.

HIV is known to progressively undermine the immune system. It does this by attacking and killing a particular group of white blood cells known as the T-helper cells. Normally the T-helper cells (also known as T4 cells) play a vital role in the prevention of infection. When an infection occurs they multiply rapidly, signalling to other parts of the body's immune system that an infection has occurred. As a result the body produces antibodies – chemical substances developed by the immune system to fight infectious agents found in the body. Apart from mobilising the body's defence systems to fend off an infection, the T-helper cells also signal to another group of white blood cells, known as T-suppressor or T8 cells, when it is time for the immune system to wind down its attack.

Normally we have more T-helper cells in the blood than T-suppressor cells, and when the immune system is functioning properly the ratio is about two to one. In people with AIDS that ratio is reversed, with T-suppressor cells outnumbering the T-helper cells. As a result, a person with AIDS not only has fewer helper cells available to ward off infection, but also they have an excess of suppressor cells which work against the helper cells carrying out their job.

Apart from knowing that it kills T-helper cells we also know that, unlike most other viruses, HIV changes the structure of the cells it attacks. It does this by incorporating its own genetic code into the genetic material of the cells it infects. The result is that when the infected cell multiplies it produces more viruses which then invade nearby T-helper cells. The process is then repeated over and over again.

Viruses which function in this way are called *retroviruses*. What makes them harder to deal with than other viruses is that because the virus becomes part and parcel of the genetic structure of the cells it infects, there is no way of getting rid of it. This means that people who are infected with the virus probably become infected for life. It also unfortunately means that a person who is infected with HIV may also be infectious for life.

The way in which the virus destroys the function of the immune system is not fully understood. One current but unproven theory is that the destruction of the immune system that occurs in people with AIDS may be due to the body recognising its own infected T-helper cells as 'the enemy'. If this were the case, then what the body's defence mechanisms might do is start producing antibodies against the infected T-cells to try and destroy them. However, antibodies would also be produced against the *uninfected* T-helper cells, possibly destroying them as well, or making them incapable of functioning properly. In this way, HIV would destroy the immune system not simply by killing off T-cells, but by tricking the body into attacking its own defence mechanisms.

HIV does not only attack the body's immune system.

Research has shown that the virus can also cause damage
to the brain and the central nervous system. Autopsies
carried out on the brains of people who have died from
AIDS have revealed that the virus can cause a massive
loss of brain tissue. At the same time, other researchers
have managed to isolate HIV from the cerebrospinal fluid
of individuals who showed no symptoms of having AIDS.
These findings are extremely disturbing. They suggest
that the effects of HIV are likely to be far worse than have
previously been imagined. Whilst researchers still
thought that HIV only attacked the immune system, all
those infected with the virus, but with no apparent
symptoms of AIDS or related illness, could be considered
to have had a lucky escape. Now, with this recent
research, the fear is that those who have been infected
with HIV might eventually suffer some kind of damage to
the brain and the central nervous system.

We don't yet fully understand all the effects HIV may
have. One of the difficulties in predicting what the long-
term effects of infection with HIV might be is that it is a
slow-working virus. People with AIDS will have been
carrying the virus around with them for some time, often
for several years, before developing symptoms of the
disease. As the first cases of AIDS were only recorded in
1981, we do not know for certain what the incubation
period is. It could be six years or longer. If the incubation
period is longer than has previously been estimated, as
many people now believe, then only in the next few years
will the full effects of HIV become known.

Where did AIDS originate?

The simple answer is that no one knows for sure. Most
people believe that the virus which can cause AIDS
probably originated in Central Africa and was exported,
via Haiti, to the United States and the rest of the world.
The reason for this is not merely that the virus is

extremely prevalent in Uganda, Zaire, Rwanda and other Central African nations. More convincing than this was the discovery that a virus very similar to the one which causes AIDS was endemic in the African green monkey. Interestingly, the virus seems to have few ill-effects in green monkeys. However, in a different species of monkey, macaques, this monkey virus causes an immunodeficiency syndrome resembling human AIDS.

Several theories have been put forward to try and account for how this monkey-AIDS virus could have found its way into humans. One suggestion is that the virus may have been transmitted as a result of people being bitten by green monkeys; another, by insects carrying the virus.

Some African critics have accused American and European researchers of being racist in their attempts to show that AIDS originated in Africa. Africans' concerns about being international scapegoats for the AIDS epidemic parallel those of the gay community in the United States. There the fear is that the association of AIDS with gay men will lead to renewed anti-gay and anti-lesbian feeling. In Africa the concerns are that 'blaming AIDS on blacks' will increase racism, both at home and abroad.

Certainly, there is no conclusive evidence linking the origin of AIDS with Africa. This is something which many African governments have been at pains to point out, some of them also denying that there is any such thing as an AIDS epidemic in Africa. There are understandable reasons why Africans should have reacted in this way. Nations with the highest reported number of AIDS cases are said to fear the economic consequences of being described as centres of AIDS infection, especially in terms of how it would affect their essential tourist industries. Kenya is a case in point. After coffee exports, tourism is Kenya's most important industry for attracting money into the country.

Apart from the link with Africa, there has been

speculation that the AIDS epidemic is the result, either deliberate or accidental, of experiments in germ warfare carried out by the CIA. Another unsubstantiated theory is that the prevalence of AIDS is related to fall-out from nuclear weapons testing. Others, like the Moral Majority in the United States, have claimed that AIDS is a punishment from God for society's 'acceptance' of homosexuality, promiscuity and prostitution.

How serious is AIDS?

Any disease which invariably results in death, and for which there is no vaccine and no known cure, is extremely serious. It becomes all the more so when it spreads rapidly.

AIDS is a new disease. The first cases were seen in the late 1970s. Since then, the illness has been diagnosed around the world with increasing frequency. By the end of October 1986 over 33,000 cases had been reported worldwide, in countries as far afield as Norway, New Zealand and Canada. In America there are over 27,000 recorded cases (November 1986).

The number of new cases of AIDS continues to rise. In the United Kingdom the first case of AIDS was reported at the end of 1981. Since then the number of cases reported has increased rapidly. For example, at the end of 1983 there were only 31 cases of AIDS recorded. Three years later this figure had risen to almost 600. However, people with AIDS represent only a tiny proportion of all those who are infected with the virus. By the end of 1986, it was estimated that between 30,000 and 40,000 people living in this country had been infected with HIV. Although some of these will not develop AIDS or HIV-related illnesses they will probably be able to transmit the virus to others who might.

It is difficult to know whether this rapid rate of infection will continue. Clearly the potential for large-scale infection is present. Some estimate there may be a million people infected with HIV, and 18,000 with AIDS, in the UK by the end of the decade. Whether this occurs or not will depend largely on the efforts that are made, both at governmental and individual levels, to prevent the transmission of HIV. In the United States the two cities with the largest numbers of AIDS cases – San Francisco and New York – appear to have levelled off in their rate of increase. However, other cities and towns, which have not been made as AIDS-aware, are still experiencing a rapid rate of increase in AIDS cases.

So what has all this got to do with women? I ask this question because until very recently AIDS tended to be seen as an issue primarily affecting gay men. The media played a significant role in constructing this view, frequently referring to AIDS as the 'gay disease' or the 'gay plague'. One effect this had was to render other groups at risk invisible, most especially women. In fact, while approximately three-quarters of those with AIDS in Europe and America are gay or bisexual men, and while in some cities such as San Francisco this percentage is much higher, a significant number of women have also developed AIDS. In the United States, for example, though very few women were affected at first, women now make up about 7 per cent of the total number of people with AIDS. It is evidence from Central Africa, however, that most seriously challenges the idea that AIDS is something women (and heterosexuals) rarely get. Studies carried out in the tropical African zone have shown that apart from infection with HIV being extremely widespread (estimates suggest that between 5 and 10 million Africans may be carrying the virus), AIDS occurs about equally in women and men. For Third World women AIDS is a major health issue. Over the next few years thousands of African women will die from it.

We are only just beginning to see cases of AIDS in women in the United Kingdom. It is therefore difficult to say how many women are likely to be affected and how quickly. It may be that the epidemic curve will follow the pattern of that for women in the United States. Alternatively, there may be differences due to the different social conditions of British and American women at risk.

In considering how serious an issue AIDS is for women it is also important to recognise that AIDS has occurred at a time when the National Health Service is severely strained in caring for the sick. In the context of the Thatcher government's policy of cutting NHS spending, this is likely to place a greater burden for AIDS care on the 'community'. In our society it has traditionally been women who have been the main providers of community care: for children, for the elderly and for the sick.

How is AIDS transmitted?

Much of the fear and panic surrounding AIDS is due to a lack of understanding of how HIV is passed from one person to another. Many people believe that it is possible to get AIDS through normal, everyday contact with people who carry the virus. This is not the case. You do not catch HIV simply by being near, eating with or touching a person who is infected by it. Nor will you catch HIV by touching objects used by someone who has the virus. No one has ever become infected through swimming in the same pool as an infected person, through sharing clothes or towels, or through drinking out of the same cup as them. HIV is very fragile and is easily killed outside the body. There is absolutely no reason to think that it can be spread through the air, or by casual social contact.

Perhaps the best evidence that the virus which can lead to AIDS is not passed on through ordinary everyday contact comes from health care workers who have been treating AIDS patients for several years. There has not been a single case of a doctor, nurse or hospital technician developing AIDS as a result of working with AIDS patients and only a few who have contracted the virus through accidentally injecting themselves. All evidence indicates that it is prefectly safe to work, play, go to school and live with people who have AIDS or are antibody positive. If HIV could be contracted through everyday contact there would by now be many reported cases of AIDS, not only among health care workers, but also among family and friends caring for people with AIDS.

In most cases of AIDS the virus was acquired sexually. You risk catching HIV by having vaginal or anal intercourse with someone who is already infected. Other ways of having sex are risky if they too involve you coming into contact with body fluids which contain HIV. These include semen, blood and vaginal secretions. Ways of reducing the risk of infection by practising safe sex are described in Chapters 3 and 4.

It is wrong to think that HIV can only be spread through gay sex. Despite the early association of AIDS with gay men, we now know that the virus can be transmitted heterosexually, both from men to women and from women to men. The most striking evidence for this is the widespread occurrence of AIDS in Central Africa, where it seems to have little to do with homosexual behaviour. At first researchers resisted a sexual explanation. One theory was that blood-sucking insects, such as mosquitoes, might carry the virus from person to person. This now seems very unlikely. HIV infection occurs mainly in women and men of reproductive age. People of all ages get bitten by insects.

Another explanation put forward was that the virus had been transmitted through doctors using the same unsterile needles on different people. This is a common practice in Africa. The use of unscreened blood donations has also been considered as a possible explanation. Undoubtedly both of these practices are ways in which HIV could be transmitted. Research suggests, however, that neither unscreened blood donations nor the use of unsterile needles is the chief means of transmission. The main way in which African women and men appear to catch the virus which can lead to AIDS is through vaginal intercourse.

In addition to being able to transmit it to their heterosexual partners, women who are infected with HIV can also pass it on to their children during pregnancy, through the placenta, at birth, or possibly through their breast milk. The relationship between pregnancy and AIDS is discussed in the next chapter. The possibility of a woman being able to transmit the virus to another woman sexually has been little talked about or researched, though we should note that lesbians are a low-risk group for sexually transmitted diseases generally. This and some of the other issues which AIDS raises for lesbians are discussed in Chapter 3.

Apart from being seen initially as a gay disease, AIDS has also been associated with promiscuity. For example, in their book *AIDS: The Deadly Epidemic*, Graham Hancock and Enver Carim state that HIV most definitely is transmitted through 'the shared use of needles by drug abusers, and promiscuous sex of any kind' – with an infected person of course – (Hancock and Carim, Gollancz, 1986).

One of the problems with this is that people may conclude not just that if they only have sex with one person they won't get AIDS, but also that everyone infected with HIV or with AIDS must have been 'promiscuous'. This is not the case. Like pregnancy, you only need to have sex once to catch the virus.

The word 'promiscuous' means different things to different people. It also means different things depending upon whether it is used about a woman or a man. As part of the sexual 'double standard' that operates in our society, it is generally more acceptable for men to have more sex with more people at all ages than it is for women. Consequently, 'casual sex' in women is seen as reprehensible in a way that it is not for men (unless they happen to be gay). This has important implications for who gets the blame for spreading AIDS. For example, it is women, as prostitutes, and not their male clients who have been singled out as important in the heterosexual transmission of HIV. (This is discussed in more detail in the following chapter.)

Hancock and Carim fail to specify what exactly *they* mean by 'promiscuous sex'. What they do say suggests that it is not so much the way you have sex that is important as the number of different people you have sex with. By implication, if you restrict your sexual activities to one person you ought to be OK.

Unfortunately, being monogamous is no protection against AIDS if your partner is infected with HIV and you engage in sexual acts that allow transmission of the virus. Also, monogamy is not a realistic choice for many people. Sexual relations end for all sorts of reasons and, as a result, people will develop new ones. Young people do not always find the 'right person' first time. Also, some may find it emotionally or economically difficult to limit sex to one person. A woman working as a prostitute, for example, would have to find an alternative way of financially supporting herself and, in many cases, her children.

Although 'promiscuity' *per se* does not cause AIDS, it may affect your chances of catching the virus which can lead to it. The more people you have sex with the more likely it is that at least one of them will be infected with HIV. This is especially true if you have sex with people from high-risk groups (for example, with people who are injecting drug users or with sexually active gay or bisexual men). Having said this, it is important to recognise that cutting down on the number of sexual partners one has will not significantly reduce the risks of catching HIV if you don't also practise safe sex. It is not primarily the number of people you have sex with that creates risk for infection with HIV, but rather what you do. Related to this, it would have been more accurate if from the beginning researchers had talked about certain kinds of sexual activity between men being high-risk, rather than just about gay or bisexual men. A lot of men have sex with other men and do not see themselves as gay or even bisexual. The danger is that, because their identity differs, they may think that what they do does not put them at risk. This will have implications for the women, as well as the men, they have sex with, a situation made worse by the fact that many men do not tell their wives or girlfriends when they have sex with another man.

HIV is passed on whenever blood from an infected person enters the body of an uninfected person. Apart from certain sexual practices which allow this to happen, the main risk is to injecting drug users who share needles, syringes or other equipment used for mixing or injecting drugs.

In the past some people were given blood or blood products which had been infected with HIV. Haemophiliacs, in particular, caught the virus this way, through treatment with the blood products factor 8 and factor 9 which help the blood to clot. Factor 8 is made from the plasma of thousands of donors. Plasma is the fluid left when the cells have been removed from the blood. Even if only one or two of these donors are infected with HIV, the chances are that the factor 8 produced from their blood will also contain the virus. In this country it is estimated that up to two-thirds of haemophiliacs may be infected with HIV. About a third of those who have so far been tested are antibody positive. Only 21 haemophiliacs have so far developed AIDS (October 1986). Fortunately, the risk of people catching the virus this way has now been largely eliminated. Since 1985, all donated blood has been tested for HIV and blood products heat treated, a simple process which kills the virus.

With rare exceptions, haemophilia occurs only in men. Very few women have therefore been at risk of contracting HIV this way. However as sexual partners of men with haemophilia they may be at risk.

Before the HIV antibody test was developed, there was

also a small risk of contracting the virus through blood transfusions. The widespread reporting of such cases in the media immediately created generalised fear and panic. Suddenly AIDS was no longer a disease of certain minority groups, it was a public health issue. Anyone might conceivably need a blood transfusion sometime in their life, and therefore anyone might conceivably catch HIV and develop AIDS. One response to this scare-mongering was a public appeal to all would-be donors from high-risk groups, urging them not to give blood. Meanwhile in America those who had the money to do so began storing their own blood in case of an emergency.

Nowadays, through the use of the HIV antibody test, blood donors are screened for infection with HIV and any blood found to be infected is rejected. As a result the risk of contracting HIV through transfusion of blood or blood products has largely been eliminated.

Unfortunately this is not the case in many Third World countries, especially African countries where the lack of effective screening of donors means that transmission of the virus through blood transfusions will continue.

It is important that people learn to recognise the risks of contracting HIV and protect themselves against them. Equally important is that people do not panic. The risk of infection with HIV for women in the United Kingdom at present is very low. In addition, not all of those who are infected with the virus develop AIDS.

Women in high-risk groups, or whose sexual partners are, need to take certain precautions, but women outside of those groups need worry very little about getting AIDS.

Who gets AIDS?

AIDS occurs most commonly among gay or bisexual men in the West. Almost three-quarters of all people with AIDS in America and a slightly greater proportion in the United Kingdom fall into this category.

In the United States the next major group are drug users who share needles, syringes or other equipment for mixing and injecting drugs. When drug users share needles blood from one user can be passed to another; if the first person has the virus it can be transmitted to the second. 'Pumping' – irrigating blood in and out of the syringe in order not to leave any of the drug behind – increases the risk of transmission

In the United Kingdom only a few drug users have so far been reported as having AIDS. (Though still small, the number of people who have got AIDS as a result of transfusion with blood products is greater. This group includes haemophiliacs.) A large number of those who inject drugs are however believed to be infected with HIV. It is therefore expected that over the next few years we will see many more cases of AIDS among injecting drug users.

Sexual partners of people who inject drugs, of haemophiliacs and of gay or bisexual men are at risk if they have sex which allows the transmission of HIV. (For a detailed account of what kinds of sex are 'unsafe' see Chapters 3 and 4.) This is also relevant to people who have lived or worked in Central Africa where AIDS is epidemic in the heterosexual community, with the disease as common in women as in men across a range of countries including Zaire, Uganda, Rwanda, Zambia and Kenya.

Because HIV is found in semen, women who use AID (artificial insemination by donor) as a means of getting pregnant may also be at risk. They may become infected with HIV if semen from an infected donor is used. This also puts any potential offspring at risk. Infants may be infected with HIV while in the womb or, possibly, at birth if the mother is infected.

It is extremely rare for women or men who do not fall into any of these risk groups to become infected with the virus which may lead to AIDS. Nevertheless, anyone who is exposed to HIV in a manner which permits its transmission risks catching it.

What are the symptoms of AIDS?

Many of the symptoms of AIDS are similar to those that occur in common illnesses such as colds, bronchitis and stomach flu. However in AIDS these symptoms are usually more severe and last for a long time.

The general symptoms of AIDS may include:

- Profound fatigue, which lasts for weeks, with no obvious cause.
- Unexplained fever, shaking chills or drenching night sweats, lasting longer than several weeks.
- Unexpected weight loss – over 10 pounds in less than two months.
- Swollen glands, especially in the neck or armpits.
- Thrush – a thick whitish coating in the mouth or throat. Thrush is a very common infection in healthy women, causing an irritating white discharge from the vagina. In men, thrush may appear as irritating white spots on the end of the penis or as a white discharge from the rectum.
- Persistent diarrhoea.
- Shortness of breath, gradually getting worse over several weeks, together with a dry, irritating cough that is not from smoking and has lasted longer than it would if it were just from a bad cold.
- New pink or purple, flat or raised blotches (usually painless) occurring anywhere on the skin, including on the mouth or the eyelids. Initially they may look like bruises, but they do not pale when pressed and do not disappear. They are usually harder than the skin around them. This is a form of skin cancer known as Kaposi's sarcoma. For reasons that are not yet fully understood, it is not a common symptom in women with AIDS.

If you have some of these symptoms don't be alarmed, it

does not mean that you must have AIDS. There can be lots of other reasons for nearly all of these symptoms. For instance, swollen glands can be a sign of glandular fever and tiredness, and fever and weight loss are much more likely to be symptoms of stress, exhaustion or of a cold coming on. If, however, you do have some of the above symptoms and think there is a possibility that you might have been infected with the virus, you should see a doctor, preferably one who is familiar with AIDS. A clinic which specialises in genito-urinary infections may be able to provide this. You can get the address of your nearest clinic by looking in the phone book under VD (venereal disease) or under STD (sexually transmitted disease). Further information about AIDS can also be obtained by contacting the Terrence Higgins Trust (see page 137).

Can AIDS be treated?

There is currently no treatment that will destroy HIV or restore the immune system. Research on antiviral drugs is being carried out in the United States, and other countries, in an attempt to provide a cure. Antiviral drugs are substances which interfere with the growth and reproduction of viruses. One problem with such drugs has been that they often do not discriminate between infected cells and healthy cells. In order to be effective an antiviral drug would need to attack only infected cells, leaving healthy cells undamaged. Another problem is that most antiviral drugs are too large to pass through into the cerebrospinal fluid or the brain, where HIV may be.

Even if an antiviral drug capable of reaching the brain and cerebrospinal fluid were developed, there would still be problems. HIV incorporates itself into the genetic code of the cells it infects. As there is no way of disentangling the virus from the genetic code of the host cells, the only means of getting rid of HIV is to kill all of the cells it has infected. This becomes very difficult once the virus has entered the brain, as it would mean killing off vital brain cells.

Some of the antiviral drugs which are being researched have prompted a temporary remission in many people with AIDS. Studies of the drug Ribavarin, for example, have shown that it can slow down production of HIV. Tests on other antiviral agents, such as Suramin, HPA-23 and Ansamycin, have also demonstrated a reduction in the amount of virus present. Unfortunately, although certain antiviral drugs may help to slow down the progress of the disease, none of the drugs tested so far looks like providing a miracle cure for AIDS. More likely, a successful cure will come from a combination of various drugs and therapies.

In addition to the antiviral drugs already being tested, research is also being carried out on drugs which influence the immune system. Some of these are immune-boosting drugs, such as Interferon. Others, like Cyclosporin, act by suppressing the immune system. This latter approach to treatment stems from the theory that HIV works by tricking the immune system into destroying itself. By slowing down the immune system some researchers believe one might also slow down or stop this process of immune self-destruction.

At the time of writing, the drug AZT (Azidothymidine), manufactured by the Wellcome drugs company, is the latest AIDS drugs hope. Whilst the drug does not get rid of the virus it has been successful in cutting death rates among some AIDS patients in the United States. It is not, however, a cure for AIDS and without further testing it is difficult to know how useful it will prove to be.

Although there is not yet a cure for AIDS, the infections and cancers associated with AIDS can be treated with varying success. These treatments include antibiotics, chemotherapy, radiation therapy and experimental techniques. Unfortunately, many of these treatments have side-effects. One of the most common illnesses found in people with AIDS is pneumocystis carinii pneumonia

(PCP). If caught early, pneumocystis can be effectively treated with antibiotics, which can have unpleasant side-effects. Nowadays doctors are trying to prevent recurrence of PCP by keeping people with AIDS on preventative antibiotics.

Another common symptom of AIDS in men is Kaposi's sarcoma. Treatment for this involves both radiation therapy and chemotherapy. Whilst in some cases this is effective, there may be side-effects such as hair loss and nausea. A further problem with one of the drugs used to treat Kaposi's sarcoma, Vinblastine, is that it suppresses the immune system. The result can be that although the cancer may be treated, the body's immunity to infection is lowered even further, allowing other life-threatening illnesses such as pneumocystis to take hold.

Despite the fact that people with AIDS are often successfully treated for specific infections, and may lead active lives for long periods of time, the harsh reality is that no one has yet been known to recover from AIDS. Most people die within two or three years of being diagnosed. Faced with this, a number of people with AIDS have rejected conventional medical treatment and have decided to try a different approach. This holistic approach to health aims to treat the 'whole person' – physically, emotionally, spiritually and mentally – by getting the body to use its natural forces to heal itself. Holistic treatment of AIDS focuses on the underlying cause of the illness, the destruction of the body's natural defence systems, and seeks to restore the immune system through alternative therapies. These include taking regular exercise, maintaining a healthy diet by cutting out things like sugar, caffeine and alcohol, vitamin therapy, stress reduction and learning to 'think positive'.

Those who follow holistic treatments experience the same sad outcome as those undergoing traditional treatment, a gradual weakening of the body and eventually death. However some people feel that holistic therapies allow them to maintain their health and a high quality of life for a longer period than would be the case if they were having chemotherapy or other medical treatments. They may feel more in control of their lives and their health. Because they encourage people's efforts to help themselves, such regimes may also give a person greater hope.

Another goal in the treatment of AIDS is the development of a vaccine that would induce lasting immunity to HIV and thus prevent AIDS. This probably won't be produced until the 1990s at the earliest. Although the development of such a vaccine is proceeding, it faces major obstacles. When a vaccine is injected into the bloodstream a small amount of the infectious agent (in this case HIV) is released, causing the body to produce antibodies against the infection. These antibodies remain in the blood ready to stop any future infection occurring. They do this by locking into the outer coat of infectious organisms, thereby rendering them harmless. One of the characteristics of HIV is that it is constantly mutating and producing different strains with different outer coatings. If the antibodies being produced no longer fit the lock on the outer coat of the virus they will be unable to do their job. Even if a vaccine is produced, therefore, it may still not offer the ultimate solution. The fact that the virus keeps changing could mean that the vaccine would quickly become ineffective against new strains of HIV. A further problem is that the antibodies produced to HIV don't actually kill the virus.

There have been encouraging reports in the last year of research being conducted in Britain. However, even if a vaccine were produced tomorrow, it would take years of development and testing before it would become widely available. Prevention may be the only effective defence against AIDS for a long time to come.

2 AIDS in women

High-risk groups

Women make up approximately 7 per cent of the total number of AIDS cases in the United States. Because this is a relatively small proportion, AIDS in women often tends to get overlooked. This is also true of the UK, where we are only just beginning to see cases of AIDS in women. The fact that in Africa thousands of women have AIDS is not the only reason why this silence needs to be challenged. In addition to those who have already developed AIDS, many more women have the virus or are concerned and worried that they might catch it. Women need to know as much as possible about AIDS and what they can do to protect themselves.

Very little research has been done on what constitutes a high-risk group of women. One study which has looked at this is the San Francisco-based community study known as AWARE (Association for Women's AIDS Research and Education). The aim of this study is to find out which groups of women are at risk for HIV infection as a result of heterosexual contact, by testing for antibodies to the virus. The women taking part in the study have either had sexual contact with, or donor insemination from, a man in an AIDS risk group (gay or bisexual man, injecting drug user, Haitian, haemophiliac or known AIDS patient) or have had multiple sexual relationships with men. For the purposes of this study this was defined as five or more sexual partners in the previous three years. Women have not been recruited for the study directly. Instead, women who feel they may be at risk are encouraged to call in and discuss their own risk situation and the project. Those who agree to take part are interviewed about sexual and lifestyle practices that are associated with AIDS, such as injecting drug use, and are given the antibody test. Preliminary reports, based on the first 220 participants, show 4 per cent to be antibody positive. Although this is too small a number to say anything very definite, when compared with those women who had a negative test result this group were more likely to have had bisexual or injecting drug-using sexual partners, or partners with AIDS. They were also much more likely to report ever injecting drugs themselves.

The largest group of women with AIDS in the United States are women who inject drugs, over half of the total. Of the rest, 27 per cent are women who have had sexual contact with men in risk groups and 10 per cent are women who have received blood transfusions. The remaining 11 per cent do not fall into any of the known risk groups. This includes women with incomplete medical histories. Also a lot of women who have developed AIDS may not wish to admit to being in a particular high-risk group. They may be too afraid or embarrassed to admit that they inject drugs, for instance, or have a boyfriend or husband who is bisexual.

The vast majority of women with AIDS are young women between 20 and 40 years old. AIDS also affects a lot more women of colour. In the United States, for example, only 26 per cent of women who have AIDS are white, 51 per cent are black and 22 per cent are hispanic. So overall 73 per cent of women with AIDS are women of colour (February 1986). This is clearly disproportionate with the percentage of the population which they

represent. According to health officials, this reflects the
more widespread use of injectable drugs among black and
hispanic women. It may also be because there is an
'African' epidemic pattern in this group.

To summarise, women are at risk of acquiring the virus
which can lead to AIDS if they:

- Inject drugs and share needles.
- Have sexual contact with, or are artificially inseminated
  by, a man who is infected with HIV.
- Receive a blood transfusion with blood infected with
  HIV. (In the UK and the United States this risk of
  infection has now been largely eliminated.)

Injecting drug users

Women who inject drugs are at risk for AIDS (and other
diseases) if they share needles, syringes or other equipment used for mixing and injecting drugs. In New York
there are 'shooting galleries', where needles and syringes
may be hired and are frequently shared by large numbers
of users. Although there is nothing to compare with this
in the UK, many drug users who inject drugs do share
needles. Unfortunately, if you inject yourself using an
unsterilised needle which has previously been used by
someone infected with HIV you could catch the virus
yourself. (In addition, sharing ear-piercing equipment
and tattooing, electrolysis and acupuncture needles may
carry some degree of risk.)

It is not only intravenous (IV) drug use which carries
this risk. Injecting yourself anywhere could lead to the
virus being passed on. Irrigating blood in and out of the
syringe in order not to leave behind any of the drug it
contains is likely to increase the chances of this
happening.

In the United States women who inject drugs run the
greatest risk of developing AIDS. By early November

1986, 1,806 women in the United States had AIDS. More than half of these were women who injected drugs. In contrast to this, there have so far been very few cases of AIDS among injecting drug users in the UK. Only two women were reported to have contracted AIDS through injecting drugs (by November 1986). Over the next few years it is likely that in the UK we will see a growing number of women who inject drugs develop AIDS or HIV-related illness.

The DHSS estimate that in England 10 per cent, on average, of those who inject drugs are already infected with HIV (November 1986). In some parts of the country this figure may be even higher. In Edinburgh, for example, studies suggest that more than 50 per cent of injecting drug users may be infected. This reflects the difficulties which those injecting drugs have had in obtaining sterile needles and syringes, causing many to risk infection with HIV by sharing their 'works' – an unfortunate consequence of police attempts to regulate drug use in Scotland by limiting the availability of hypodermic needles.

Drug use puts women directly at risk where they themselves inject drugs and share dirty and possibly infected needles. As sexual partners of men who inject drugs women are also at risk. As I have already mentioned, the virus can be transmitted from a man to a woman during vaginal intercourse. Women who make love with men who inject drugs should therefore practise 'safe sex'. (A full discussion of what is safe and what is risky sex is provided in Chapter 4.) Women who inject drugs may also be at risk of HIV infection through sex if they use prostitution as a means of financing their drug addiction.

Drug users who are antibody positive have sometimes been denied surgical operations, dental treatment and other forms of medical care, including treatment for their drug problems. Such unsympathetic treatment stems in part from the anxiety which some health workers have that they may contract HIV from patients who are infected with the virus. It may also be related to the assumption that drug users get what they deserve because they use drugs. Gay men have also been subjected to similar kinds of injustice. In their case, however, it is homophobic beliefs that homosexuality is abnormal, sick or morally wrong that have led some to make the frighteningly insensitive claim that AIDS is no more than what they deserve.

Whilst the virus must be present in the body for AIDS to occur, infection with HIV does not necessarily lead to the development of AIDS or HIV-related illness. It is possible that other as yet unknown factors, which also affect the immune system, may play a part in determining who goes on to develop AIDS once they have been infected with HIV. Drug users use substances which suppress the immune system. Whilst there is no evidence that drug use is a co-factor, researchers believe that this may increase the chances of those infected with HIV developing AIDS. Poor nutrition has also been suggested as a possible co-factor. Where there is an association between drug taking and eating disorders, as often seems to be the case in women, there may therefore be a further risk.

One way of avoiding these risks is to stop using drugs. For many women this will be very hard to do, but some do manage to stop with the help and support of others. If you are thinking about coming off drugs there are a number of organisations which you could contact to help you (see page 138).

A very effective way of reducing the risks of contracting HIV and possibly developing AIDS if you don't feel able to give up is not to inject. If you stop injecting drugs you are completely safe from catching the virus through taking drugs. You cannot get HIV from sniffing, snorting, smoking or swallowing drugs. There are other reasons for stopping injecting besides AIDS. Hepatitis, blood poisoning, thrombosis and nerve damage are some of the other health problems associated with injecting drugs.

If coming off or changing the way you use drugs are choices you don't feel able to make then you should stop sharing needles. This applies whether you inject drugs regularly or only occasionally, and is something that everyone can do. Since people may transmit the virus without showing any symptoms, sharing needles with someone who appears healthy is not a safeguard.

It may help to label or mark your works so that both you and other people know which are yours. Care should also be taken not to mix your gear up in a spoon or mixing bowl used by other people. When you have used a needle and syringe, bend back the needle and dispose of it safely. Do not leave used needles lying around where people can accidentally stab themselves or where others might find and use them. If you are going to re-use needles you should wash needles and syringes with bleach or alcohol after each use, leaving them to soak in alcohol until the next use. (You must get rid of all the bleach solution from the works before you re-use them.)

It is essential that women who inject drugs have access to information and advice about AIDS. This is especially true of adolescents who, if they are to become aware of the risks associated with experimenting with injectable drugs, must be given information about AIDS and how it is spread. Apart from public education campaigns, which should include guidelines for both safer sex and safer drug use, counselling and advisory services are needed. These should provide advice to women about how to reduce the risk of HIV infection to themselves and, if they are already infected, to others. Some women may also be anxious to know whether or not they came into contact with HIV whilst they were injecting drugs and will need counselling about whether or not they should take the antibody test.

Half the difficulty with AIDS prevention is getting the message across. This will not be easy with drug users who may already be at risk of early death through injecting drugs or when the advice that is being offered goes against a person's social customs. Partly for this reason, preventing the sharing of equipment may be the quickest and most effective means of limiting the spread of HIV among injecting drug users. Acknowledging this, some doctors have adopted the policy of supplying sterile needles and syringes on an exchange basis, a clean set being given only on return of the old one. Another way one might reduce the sharing of equipment, at least among some users, would be to prescribe the non-injectable drug methadone as a substitute for heroin.

Sexual transmission

Although it has probably played a limited role in the spread of AIDS in Europe and the United States to date, heterosexual transmission of HIV is possible.

In Australia, in 1985, reports that four women had been infected with HIV as a result of being artificially inseminated with semen from an infected donor provided convincing evidence of male to female transmission. Similarly, in the United States and Europe sexual transmission has occurred from men, particularly injecting drug users, to their female partners.

Evidence of sexual transmission of the virus from women to men is more sketchy. We know that HIV is present in the vaginal and cervical fluids of infected women and that, under certain conditions, sexual transmission of the virus from women to men can occur. In one case a woman who had received a kidney transplant from an HIV-infected kidney donor passed the virus on to her husband who was at no other apparent risk of infection. Several cases have also been reported where men appear to have got AIDS from sexual contact with women who inject drugs. It is not clear whether these men contracted HIV, which led to their developing AIDS, from blood associated with sex or from vaginal secretions.

Many researchers believe that the virus is less easily transmitted from a woman to a man than the other way around. Such claims are largely based on the number of reported cases, rather than on any direct evidence comparing rates of infection among the sexual partners of HIV-infected women with those of HIV-infected men. In the United States, for example, sex with a woman infected with HIV has been strongly implicated as the source of AIDS in 524 men (November 1986). This number represents only 2 per cent of all AIDS cases in men in the United States. By contrast, the number of women thought to have contracted HIV and developed AIDS through sexual contact with a man was 486, 27 per cent of the total number of women with AIDS. What this indicates is that whilst heterosexual contact has to date been relatively unimportant in the spread of AIDS among men, in women it is a significant risk factor.

The actual mechanism by which the virus gets into a woman's bloodstream, and the relative efficiency for male-female and female-male transmission, is not known. The virus might enter the bloodstream through ulcerations or erosions of the cervix or through the vaginal walls which become swollen with blood during sexual arousal. Cuts or sores on a woman's genital area may also allow semen carrying the virus to reach the bloodstream. For this reason the virus may be acquired more easily by women who have venereal infections, such as herpes or gonorrhoea.

The virus may also be transmitted more easily by women with infections which cause a discharge containing virus-infected cells. Because the virus is also found in blood, HIV may also be present in the vagina in greater quantities during a woman's period. As with male-female transmission, the virus may be passed more easily from a woman to a man if there are cuts or abrasions on the penis which would allow the virus more direct access to the bloodstream.

Apart from not knowing how the virus actually gets

into a woman's bloodstream during sex, there are also many unanswered questions about the relative risk that different sexual activities may carry. Some practices are thought to transmit the virus more readily than others. Anal intercourse often causes tearing of tissue and, some experts believe, may allow more of the virus in semen to enter the bloodstream directly. But vaginal intercourse is clearly the source of infection in many women.

Whether the virus can be transmitted orally, either by oral-genital or oral-anal contact, is not clear. (There is no evidence to suggest oral transmission through kissing.) One of the difficulties in trying to study this is that people who have oral sex very often also engage in other kinds of sex which would allow transmission of the virus such as, for instance, vaginal intercourse.

Whatever the mode of transmission is, it is clear that the proportion of women who have got AIDS through heterosexual contact is growing. As of May 1986, there were 1,304 women with AIDS in the United States. Approximately 18 per cent of these probably got AIDS through heterosexual contact. These are women who deny belonging to any known AIDS risk group, but who say that they have had sex with a man who either has AIDS or is in a high-risk group for AIDS. By early November 1986, 27 per cent of women with AIDS in the US fell into this category. When added to a proportion, as is likely, of the substantial number of women for whom, for a variety of reasons, there is no known risk factor, it is clear that, in the United States at least, a considerable number of women are getting AIDS through sexual contact with men. (In Central Africa heterosexual contact is considered to be the main way in which women get AIDS.)

In Britain, where we are only just beginning to see cases of AIDS in women, nine out of the 17 cases to date have been attributed to heterosexual contact (October 1986). A similar pattern to that in America may emerge as more women who have been infected with HIV develop AIDS. The women at risk are sexual partners of men who inject drugs and of gay or bisexual men, haemophiliacs, and men who have lived or worked in Central Africa or Haiti. The other group who are potentially at risk are women who have sex with many different men, particularly if they don't know much about them and engage in 'unsafe' sex.

Sexual partners of men at risk

Women who are sexual partners of men with AIDS, or men who are at risk of acquiring the syndrome, are themselves at risk. In the case of women who have sexual contact with men being treated for haemophilia, the risk of infection with HIV (compared to other risk factors) seems to be fairly low. Studies both in the UK and in the United States suggest that only about 10 per cent of women with male partners who have been infected with HIV through receiving treatment with factor 8 are likely to be antibody positive themselves. To further reduce the risk of infection care should be taken to make love in ways that are 'safe'.

Women can also catch the virus that can lead to AIDS through sexual contact with men who inject drugs. Of the women in the United States who have got AIDS through sex with men, the majority had partners who were injecting drug users. The next largest group were female partners of bisexual men.

The potential for transmission of HIV from bisexual men to their female sexual partners is one of the few areas where research related to women and AIDS is going on. At the University of California, Berkeley, Nancy Padian is conducting a study of bisexual men living in the San Francisco Bay area. In this study bisexual men who have tested positive on the HIV antibody test are being contacted and asked to name their female sexual contacts. These women are then traced and, if they agree to take part in the study, are given the antibody test. A similar study involving the partners of bisexual men is being carried out at the Middlesex Hospital, London.

Because they represent a possible chain of infection from gay men to the wider heterosexual community, bisexual men have had a great deal of hostility directed at them. What we should also remember, of course, is that a considerable number of men who consider themselves gay have sex with women from time to time.

Criticisms of bisexuality have not just come from the heterosexual world. Among lesbians there is concern that bisexual women may introduce AIDS into the lesbian community. This, and some of the other issues which AIDS raises for lesbians, are discussed in more detail in the following chapter.

For women it seems there is a greater risk of getting AIDS through steady sexual relationships with men who are infected with HIV than there is through having many different partners. (This may reflect the current low level of HIV infection among heterosexual men, at least in Europe and the United States.) For example, in one case where a 71-year-old woman developed AIDS, her only apparent risk factor was infrequent sexual intercourse with her husband, a 74-year-old haemophiliac who had received factor 8 concentrate. This woman had sex only with her husband, to whom she had been married for more than fifty years. Apart from demonstrating that AIDS can occur in the elderly as well as in young people, what this suggests is that even if you have sex only occasionally or with just one person, it is still possible to get AIDS if your partner is infected with HIV.

The more people you have sex with the more likely it is that at least one of them will be carrying the virus. For this reason women who have sex with many different men, whether for payment or not, are also at risk. Another kind of risk assessment is concerned with the kind of sexual practices you engage in. You are most at risk of catching the virus if you have vaginal or anal intercourse, especially if your male partner does not use a condom.

Among the first 220 participants of the San Francisco-based AWARE study, over half of the women said that they had had anal intercourse with one or more men; 50 per cent of women in the sex industry and 58 per cent of women not in the sex industry. However, half of the former group reported using protection, compared to only 12 per cent of women not in the sex industry. In general, women working as prostitutes reported more use of barrier protection methods for all types of sexual behaviour. Nevertheless, the proportion of women found to be positive on repeated tests for antibodies to HIV was the same for both groups: 4 per cent.

These findings, though preliminary, provide a useful introduction to the more general issue of prostitution and AIDS.

Prostitutes

Although there are, in 1986, nearly 2,000 women in the United States with AIDS and thousands more in Central Africa, very little research has been done on who, among women, is likely to get AIDS and how. Some high-risk groups of women have been identified, such as women who inject drugs, but others such as prostitutes are being named regardless of the fact that so far there is little direct evidence that they are a risk group.

Only one woman out of a sample of 50 prostitutes attending the genito-urinary clinic at St Mary's Hospital, London, had antibodies to HIV, and she was an injecting drug user. In West Germany, only 1 per cent of the 4,000 registered prostitutes who were tested in 1985 were antibody positive and almost all of these were heroin addicts. In San Francisco, only 4 per cent of the prostitutes taking part in the AWARE study were antibody positive. This group were much more likely to have a history of injecting drugs.

Studies such as these suggest that in the West unless a

prostitute injects drugs she is unlikely to be infected with HIV. Some women who are 'on the game' use prostitution as a way of getting drugs or money to pay for drugs. In New York, for instance, injecting drugs is reported to be widespread among the group of prostitutes known as 'streetwalkers'. These are women who pick up their clients out on the street rather than through, say, an escort agency. As a high proportion, some estimate as many as half, of the city's injecting drug users are believed to be infected with the virus, this may explain why many prostitutes in New York, and cities like it, are reported to be at risk.

Such claims need to be understood in relation to beliefs about both prostitution and AIDS. To be a prostitute is to belong to a normally despised category of women which (like homosexuality) has been linked with disease and contagion. The image of a woman who sells sex for money is often that of someone who is unclean and spreads infection and is immoral. During the hunt for the Yorkshire Ripper, Peter Sutcliffe, for example, both the police and the press sought to make a distinction between the killing of 'innocent' women and the killing of prostitutes.

AIDS has often been talked about, especially by certain sections of the mass media, in a way that is equally judgmental. The assumption that AIDS is the result of bad behaviour pervades the perception of it as a disease transmitted by, presumably guilty, carriers such as homosexuals, drug users and prostitutes, to 'innocent victims', such as haemophiliacs, receivers of blood transfusions and infants. In this view it is the actions of certain groups of people that cause AIDS, not a virus.

Initially, it was gay men who were blamed for AIDS. This ensured that gay men who got AIDS, of which there have been a great many, received little public sympathy. Not only was it seen as their own fault that they had become ill but also, and of far more interest to the heterosexual majority, it was perceived as their fault that those who were not gay developed AIDS. Homosexuals were judged to be guilty of spreading the disease to others.

With the growing recognition that AIDS is not a 'gay disease' and can be transmitted heterosexually, a new scapegoat became necessary. Women prostitutes apparently fitted the bill nicely. This has been especially true in Africa, where prostitutes have been blamed for the rapid spread of infection in a number of Central African countries. Similarly, in the UK and in the United States the association of prostitutes with the spread of AIDS gave right-wing moralists another reason to condemn prostitution as 'morally wrong.'

Although studies in the United States and Europe have shown that some prostitutes, mainly those who inject drugs, are carrying the virus, few if any cases of AIDS in men can be unequivocally linked to them. Of the men in the United States who have AIDS only about 5 per cent do not fall into any of the known risk groups (i.e. are not gay or bisexual, injecting drug users, haemophiliacs or men who have had a blood transfusion). That some of these men say they have a history of visiting prostitutes is difficult to interpret. A lot of men who have got AIDS may not wish to admit to being in a particular high-risk group. Indeed, given that it is generally seen as both more understandable and more acceptable for a man to pay a woman to have sex with him than it is for a man to desire another man, some men may claim to have got the virus from a prostitute because it is much less difficult than saying that they are bisexual or gay.

The possibility that a prostitute might catch HIV from a customer, though rarely discussed, is something many prostitutes are afraid of. Leading AIDS experts advise against sexual contact with men in the known risk groups. Those women who, like prostitutes, are not always in a position to be able to follow this advice should practise safe sex to reduce their risk of infection. The problem with this is that a man may take the view that if he has paid for sex he's entitled to have the kind of sex he wants. Many men, for instance, don't like using condoms and may refuse to wear one. Some prostitutes may agree to this, even though it puts them at risk, as not to do so would mean a reduction in their earnings. This is likely to be especially true of the many women for whom prostitution is an alternative to poverty.

Those who regard prostitutes as responsible for the spread of AIDS tend to ignore men's involvement in prostitution. This has happened before. In the mid-nineteenth century concerns about the incidence of venereal disease among British soldiers led to the passing of the Contagious Diseases Acts. Under the terms of these Acts it was women suspected of being prostitutes, and not soldiers, who were required to register and have regular medical examinations. The Acts were vigorously opposed by feminists like Josephine Butler as clearly unfair to women. They upheld a sexual double standard, which still exists today, by seeking to regulate women while ignoring men's role in the spread of venereal disease.

In much the same way it is prostitutes and not their male clients who are now being blamed for the spread of AIDS. Again the concern is that this may lead to new forms of social control of women. With the introduction of blood testing for infection by HIV, the possibility of introducing registration and compulsory screening of prostitutes obviously exists. Similarly, the government might allow the use of quarantine to isolate women with HIV or AIDS whom, it might be feared, might continue to work as prostitutes.

This is perhaps not as far-fetched as it might seem. Some MPs, concerned about AIDS, have already called for brothels to be made legal, on the grounds that prostitutes could then be officially registered and required to submit to regular health checks. Legislation already exists in Britain to allow local authorities to keep a person with AIDS in hospital if it is considered that they are a risk to others. As yet there have been no reports of prostitutes being subject to such legal regulation; but then there are very few women in Britain who, so far, have developed AIDS.

Rape

The fear of being raped is a form of male oppression all women share. It is something which, in countless ways, shapes our daily lives: whether we feel able to go out alone, especially at night; whether we feel dependent on a man for protection; whether we feel we could ever live alone. Recent statistics on sexual violence towards women confirm that this is a well-founded fear. In 1985, in England and Wales, there were more than 11,000 cases of indecent assault on women reported and 1,842 cases of rape (Home Office figures). These figures take no account of the sexual violence which goes unreported, or of the occurrence of rape within marriage as, according to British law, it is impossible for a woman to be raped by her husband. The law further ignores women's experience of sexual violence by limiting its definition of rape to penetration of the vagina by a penis. Other forms of sexual violence, such as forced oral sex or anal intercourse, or the insertion of bottles, sticks or other objects into the vagina, however violent or humiliating, are not rape. For the many women who have encountered sexual violence at some point in their lives, rape is the experience of being forced, against their will, to engage in sexual' acts, which may include vaginal intercourse.

With AIDS, the fear of being raped takes on a new dimension. The rapist may be infected with HIV which may be transmitted during forced intercourse with a woman. The more violent the attack the more likely it is that a woman will suffer internal bruising, lacerations and bleeding. This may make it easier for the virus to enter the bloodstream.

In some cases sexual violence against women leads to their death either from suicide, as a result of the emotional trauma caused by the attack, or from the physical injuries directly inflicted on them. Now there is a further possibility to consider: AIDS.

African women

In early 1983, doctors in Brussels and Paris reported AIDS-like illnesses among people without any known lifestyle risk factors for AIDS. A high proportion of these were Africans and Europeans who had been living in Zaire or Rwanda. More than anything else it was the subsequent discovery that AIDS was widespread in Central Africa which challenged the view that AIDS was a 'gay disease'; something women and heterosexuals rarely got.

In Africa women make up approximately half of the known number of AIDS cases. Many of these women are natives of Zaire or other Central African countries such as Kenya, Rwanda and Uganda, where AIDS is known locally as 'slim disease' because of its association with weight loss.

It is difficult to estimate how many African women are affected. Many African governments have been reluctant to report their AIDS cases, some denying that there is any such thing as an AIDS epidemic in Africa. African reactions of this kind are understandable when one considers the effects such claims are having on Africa's tourist industries. There is also concern that associating Africa with AIDS will lead to increased racism, both at home and abroad, a concern which has been strengthened by attempts to show that AIDS originated in Africa.

The number of African women with AIDS, or who have been infected with HIV, is thought to be high. Several studies carried out in some African cities and rural areas suggest that as many as one in ten may have the virus. Apart from being extremely widespread (some estimate that between 5 and 10 million Africans living in the central tropical zone may now be infected with HIV), women and men appear to be affected in equal numbers. Why are so many more women getting AIDS in Africa than in either Europe or the United States?

In general, transmission of HIV within Africa is less well understood than in other countries. Most Africans, both women and men, deny either injecting drugs or homosexual activity. Similarly, although some cases of AIDS have resulted from blood transfusions, the majority of African people with AIDS deny exposure to blood products. The suggestion that blood-sucking insects such as mosquitoes might be responsible for carrying the virus from person to person is now thought to be highly unlikely. AIDS occurs mainly in people who are sexually active and who live in urban, not rural districts.

Another explanation put forward is that the use of unsterilised syringes and needles for injecting vaccines and medicines may have led to the rapid spread of AIDS. This is a common practice in Africa, especially in the poorer areas where one needle might be used to inject dozens of people. Undoubtedly the virus is passed on in this way, as it is through unscreened blood donations. (Transmission would also be possible through non-sterile instruments used for tattooing, ritual scarification, ear-piercing, circumcision, clitoridectomy and infibulation.) However, it is generally believed that in Africa the main way in which AIDS is spread is by heterosexual activity.

Anal intercourse, perhaps practised as a method of contraception, might explain the high rate of HIV infection. (Anal intercourse may also occur as a result of cultural taboos about having vaginal sex whilst a woman is menstruating.) Unfortunately, we lack information about what kinds of sexual practices are common among Africans. What most people say is that they don't have anal sex. This is not surprising. People are unlikely to

want to admit they do things which are heavily stigmatised in their culture. Likewise, most Africans deny
having oral sex or oral-anal contact. It is in the light of
this, rather than of any detailed research on the rates of
transmission associated with different sex acts, which in
any case would be extremely difficult to carry out, that
vaginal intercourse has come to be regarded as a major
risk factor for African women.

It is important to remember that in Africa, the world's
poorest continent, many women are undernourished and
in ill-health and consequently have suppressed immune
systems. If co-factors are involved in the development of
AIDS this may be a further risk factor. Also, the chances
of a woman getting the virus are likely to be enhanced by
the fact that in Africa sexually transmitted diseases are
widespread. A woman who has a sexually transmitted
infection such as gonorrhoea, for example, may have
genital sores or ulcers which could make it easier for the
virus to enter her bloodstream during intercourse. She
may also have open wounds as a result of clitoridectomy
and infibulation which are practised on some African
women. Again, this would allow easier transmission of
semen containing the virus.

The infections that a woman with AIDS will get will to
some extent reflect the organisms already present in her
body. These will vary according to where she has lived
and the kind of life she has led. In the United States and
Europe, for instance, about half of all those who have
AIDS develop pneumocystis carinii pneumonia. This does
not appear to be a common infection in African women
with AIDS; more likely they will develop reactivated
infections such as tuberculosis.

Having many different sexual partners has also been
suggested as a particular risk factor. This is a feature of
African city life, but more especially among middle-class
African men. Despite this, it is women's so-called
'promiscuous' behaviour, not men's, which has attracted
most attention. In Africa, as elsewhere, it is women

working as prostitutes who have been singled out and blamed for the spread of infection. As I indicated earlier, such a view ignores the fact that prostitution is a response to the demands of men and their sexuality.

In contrast to the United States and Europe, where it seems that unless a prostitute injects drugs infection with HIV is unusual, a large proportion of prostitutes in Central Africa are thought to be carrying the virus. In one study of Rwandan prostitutes living in the town of Butare 29 of the 33 women tested had antibodies to the virus. Following on from this it has been suggested, though not proven, that many men who are infected with HIV are likely to have caught the virus from prostitutes. There is another way of looking at this. Since the virus can be transmitted to women through sexual contact with HIV-infected men, prostitutes could be infected by their male customers – a possibility which many prostitutes fear.

Clearly AIDS is a major issue for African women. Over the next few years thousands of African women will die from it and many more will become ill. Many of the children born to women with AIDS, or who are infected with HIV, will also die. The proportion of children with AIDS is already higher in Africa than anywhere else in the world.

This situation will not change unless efforts are made to try and control the spread of the disease. Rather than seeking to pin the blame on someone (in Africa it is prostitutes, in America it is gay men), what is needed is that governments act quickly by adopting a widescale policy of AIDS prevention through major educational and public information programmes. In Africa this is made difficult by a lack of resources, and personnel, to implement such programmes. Also, in Africa poor basic facilities and health care are encouraging the spread of AIDS. The health services are ill-equipped to deal with such an epidemic. There are not the resources, for instance, to routinely screen blood donors, as is done in Europe and America, which means that HIV infection through transfusions will continue. As the social and economic consequences of the AIDS crisis in Africa become more apparent, it is only to be hoped that other countries will support the development of health and educational services within Africa aimed at controlling the spread of the disease.

Haitian women

A small but significant number of those with AIDS are Haitian women and men who apparently do not fall into any known risk group. In the United States, where many Haitian immigrants live, 249 of the more than 6,000 cases of AIDS reported by October 1984 were Haitians.

It is not known why people of Haitian descent in Haiti, the United States, Canada and Europe are getting AIDS. Homosexuality, injecting drug use and blood products do not appear to play major roles in the spread of AIDS among Haitians, although the strong social stigma attached to homosexuality within the Haitian community makes it difficult to know how common homosexual behaviour is amongst Haitian men.

One suggestion is that the virus may be transmitted through sharing needles. It is a common cultural practice of Haitians, both those living in Haiti and those who have migrated to the large urban centres in the United States, to inject medicinal agents. The needles used in these practices are frequently re-used without being sterilised, which could allow the virus to be passed from one person to another. Alternatively, others have speculated that only a small section of the Haitian population is really at risk, and that this risk is due not to practices which are widespread amongst Haitians but rather to injecting drug use, homosexuality, prostitution or some other, as yet unidentified, mode of transmission.

It was this inability to explain why Haitians get AIDS that led to their being categorised as a high-risk group.

What this implied was that it was something about Haitians, or their lifestyle, which put them at risk. This connection between AIDS and Haitians was also strengthened by the common, though unsubstantiated, belief that AIDS originated in Africa and spread to the rest of the world via Haiti. It is argued that Haitians, working in Zaire and subsequently returning home, exported the virus to Haiti, where visiting American tourists, most especially gay men, became infected. Such associations have been strongly resisted by Haitians themselves, who have condemned as racist the belief that AIDS is a Haitian disease. Certainly within the United States one consequence of classifying Haitians as high-risk for AIDS was an enhancement of the social and economic discrimination that many Haitians already faced. The Haitian government, concerned also about effects of such claims on Haiti's important tourist industry, demanded that Haitians be removed from the official list of groups at risk. This was finally achieved in 1985, when the Centers for Disease Control in Atlanta, Georgia dropped Haitians from their list of risk groups.

Their action is supported by studies of the presence of HIV among Haitians. Unlike other high-risk groups such as sexually active gay men, the rate of infection among the Haitian population is low. This suggests that simply being Haitian, in isolation from other risk factors, does not increase the risk of being infected with HIV.

Blood transfusions

Very few people have got AIDS through blood transfusions. In the United States over 27,000 cases of AIDS have been reported to the Centers for Disease Control in Atlanta (November 1986). Only 2 per cent of these were recipients of blood transfusions.

Though the risk is still low, this figure is higher for women. As of November 1986, 1,806 women in the United

States had AIDS. Of these about 10 per cent had developed the disease following transfusion with blood or plasma which had been infected with HIV. In the UK three women have been reported as having got AIDS this way (by this date).

Despite this, some women may be worried about the possibility of getting AIDS through blood transfusions. This is perhaps not surprising given what they may have heard or read about AIDS. The widespread and, very often, sensationalised coverage of such cases by certain sections of the media has greatly exaggerated the risk of developing AIDS through transfusion. As a result of the introduction of screening procedures by blood banks, the chances of contracting HIV in this way in future are *extremely* small. If a transfusion is medically necessary the risks of not getting the transfusion are much higher than the risk of getting AIDS from the transfusion.

Some women may also be worried about giving blood, in case it puts them at risk of getting AIDS through shared needles. The process of giving blood is not and never has been risky. All the equipment at blood donation centres is sterilised and used once only.

Before the introduction of screening procedures people were asked not to donate blood if they belonged to a high-risk group. As this mainly applied to men one suggestion put forward was that women only should be donors. The problem with this is that women can also carry the virus. Another suggestion was that people could store their own blood until such time as they needed it. Again such a scheme would be impractical on a wide scale, not least because of what it would cost to run.

From October 1985, with the aim of making blood transfusions as safe as possible, the National Blood Transfusion Service made it compulsory for all would-be donors to take the HIV antibody test. (In view of the fact that the test occasionally produces false negatives, those in recognised risk groups are still being advised not to give blood.) Any blood found to be infected with HIV is rejected. Unfortunately this is not the case everywhere. In Africa the lack of effective screening of donors means that the transmission of HIV through blood transfusions will continue to occur.

One possible consequence of routinely testing would-be blood donors for antibodies to HIV, is that some people might discover that they have been infected with the virus who would otherwise not have done. For most people this will be frightening news, and they will need access to support and counselling about what a positive test result means. Fortunately, the chances of this happening are extremely small. In the first six months during which it introduced screening the National Blood Transfusion Service tested over 845,000 women and men, all of whom had been asked not to give blood if they were in a high-risk group. Out of these 845,000 only 16 were confirmed as antibody positive, and most of these were subsequently found to have been at risk either through injecting drug use or gay male sex.

So, *unless* you or your sexual partner belong to a high-risk group there is no reason to fear finding out that you have the virus which can lead to AIDS, and it is safe to give blood.

Pregnancy

It is estimated that over 1,000 women of childbearing age in the United Kingdom may be infected with HIV (November 1986). Not all of these will either want or be able to have children. However for those who do desire motherhood the risks of pregnancy, both to themselves and to their potential offspring, need explaining.

It is thought that antibody positive women who become pregnant may be at greater risk of developing AIDS. More research needs to be done on this to determine how likely it is that this may happen and why. Hormonal changes that occur during pregnancy, or the fact that in a pregnant woman the immune system is suppressed to stop the body rejecting the foetus, have been suggested as possible explanations of why this may be the case. Alternatively, it could be due to the immune system becoming activated at some stage in the pregnancy, in response to the 'foreign' tissue the foetus represents.

If you are in a high-risk group and are considering pregnancy, or if you find out that you are pregnant, it is important to consider taking the antibody test. However you should only take the test after a full discussion of what the test result means and the implications that may follow from a positive result. This will include being told that there is a high chance that the virus will be passed on to any children you might have.

How this occurs is not entirely clear. At first it was thought that the virus was probably transmitted through the baby coming into contact with the mother's blood at or around the time of birth. Now we know that a pregnant woman who is infected with HIV can transmit it to the foetus. In one case cells infected with HIV were found in the tissues of a child born by caesarean section at 28 weeks to a woman who died of AIDS a few hours afterwards. The child also died three weeks later. Since the child was born by caesarean section and had no contact with his mother after delivery, this strongly suggests that the virus was passed on from mother to baby during pregnancy, via the placenta.

How likely this is is also not clear. From the studies that have so far been done it is thought that there is a relatively high risk of an infected mother giving birth to an infected child. It also seems likely that a high proportion of these infected babies will go on to develop AIDS or HIV-related disease. Many quickly become sick and, in addition to immune problems, may suffer damage to the brain and the nervous system. The risks to babies born to women who have already developed AIDS or AIDS-related illness are thought to be even greater.

This very high rate of progression to AIDS in babies

born to virus-carrying women and women with AIDS may reflect rapid production of HIV due to T-cell activation. It is now thought that T-cell activation may be necessary for the development of AIDS, insofar as the virus may only be capable of attacking and reproducing itself in activated T-helper cells and not resting ones. In young children T-cell activation is a normal part of the development of their immune system.

The number of infants with AIDS is extremely small relative to the total number of people with AIDS. By November 1986, the United States had reported only 376 cases of AIDS in children out of a total of 27,254. Similarly, in Britain AIDS in infants accounts for only about 1 per cent of all reported cases. This may change, of course, as the number of women who have been infected with HIV gradually increases.

Women carrying the virus who are considering pregnancy or are already pregnant need to be aware of one other possible risk of infection to their potential offspring. The virus is found in breast milk. The presence of the virus in a bodily fluid or tissue does not necessarily mean that it can cause an infection in another person. HIV has been found in saliva. However, there is no evidence that saliva has ever transmitted the virus. With breast milk it does seem that transmission might be possible. This follows the reporting of the case of a woman who gave birth to a child by caesarean section. The woman, because of blood loss during the operation, was given a blood transfusion after the delivery. The baby, a boy, survived and was subsequently breastfed by her. Later it was discovered that the blood used in the transfusion had been donated by someone who had since gone on to develop AIDS. Both mother and baby were tested and found to have antibodies to HIV. As the mother was apparently infected after delivery, transmission of the virus to the child could not have occurred at birth or during the pregnancy. The most likely explanation was that the child had been infected with HIV through the mother's milk. For this reason women who are infected with HIV or who fall into a high-risk group for infection are advised to bottle feed rather than breastfeed their infants.

It has also been recommended that they do not give milk to milk banks. Hundreds of hospitals run baby milk banks. Women who produce more milk than their own babies need are asked to bottle the surplus, which is then given to premature babies whose mothers are unable to produce milk. The Department of Health is considering screening women who donate milk in the same way that blood donors are screened.

Because of the possible risks to both mother and baby, advice about the relationship between pregnancy and AIDS should be available to all women at risk of infection with HIV. Apart from public education campaigns, there is a need for well-informed and sensitive counselling services for women infected with HIV who are considering pregnancy or are already pregnant. Similarly, women who are themselves healthy but have passed the virus on to their child are also likely to need the help and support of others in dealing with their feelings, very often, of guilt.

Most importantly, a woman should be able to talk to someone whom she feels is sympathetic and has an understanding of what she is going through. It's also important that counselling includes adequate and comprehensive advice about contraception and abortion. However this will only be useful if women also have access to them.

It is the medical profession which, to a large extent, controls women's access to contraception and abortion. Many doctors believe that wanting a baby is normal, instinctive and desirable in women, especially if they are married. Such beliefs have an important influence on medical practice, and can lead to a woman finding it difficult to get an abortion or certain forms of contraception. In the case of women who are infected with HIV, the medical advice is, don't have children. Where a woman who is infected with the virus is already pregnant, the recommendation is that she be considered for, and counselled about, an abortion. For some women deciding not to have a child, whether this involves having an abortion or not, will be emotionally, if not practically, difficult. This is especially likely where a woman regards becoming a mother as an important aspect of how she sees herself and her future, a view which society strongly encourages in the importance it places on women wanting and being able to have children, especially if they are married.

Apart from influencing how a woman who is infected with HIV may feel about 'choosing' not to have children, the pressures on women to become mothers may also affect the spread of AIDS. Women who want to get pregnant, unless they are using artificial insemination, will be engaging in vaginal intercourse. If either the woman or her male partner is infected with HIV then transmission of the virus to the uninfected partner may occur.

Remember, we are talking specifically about women who are either infected with HIV or who are at risk of infection. The risk of infection with this virus for women in the UK *at present* is very low.

Artificial insemination

Heterosexual intercourse, though the most common method, is not the only way of getting pregnant. Each year several thousand babies are born as a result of artificial insemination by donor (AID). The reasons why women use artificial insemination vary. Some women use this method because they can't get pregnant by their partner. Others, who are not in a steady relationship, may feel that the time is right for them to have a child on their own. Artificial insemination has also been used by lesbians who wish to conceive a child without having sex with a man. Although this might sound strange to some, wanting to have sex with someone and wanting to have a child can be quite separate desires. Another reason why some lesbians may prefer to have an AID baby is to try to ensure undisputed guardianship and custody of their child. This is very understandable given the court's reluctance to grant custody, and sometimes access, to lesbian mothers.

With artificial insemination, a syringe and not a penis is used to introduce sperm deep into a woman's vagina. This is done around the time when a woman is ovulating. The whole procedure is simple, and some women carry it out themselves without the help of doctors or an official donor organisation. In this case the term self-insemination is used.

In recent years some lesbians, and other women who are interested in becoming pregnant through artificial insemination, have become concerned about the possibility of getting AIDS. In November 1984, following publicity about AIDS, all artificial insemination clinics in Australia were closed. This decision was controversial, not only because artificial insemination was regarded as an important service for many infertile heterosexual couples, but also because there were no reported cases of AIDS due to AI. In 1985, however, four Australian women who had been artificially inseminated were found to have antibodies to HIV. They had all been inseminated with semen from a donor who was subsequently found to be infected with the virus.

This resulted in many clinics having to discard samples of donated sperm, where past donors could not be located and tested for infection with HIV. This is a procedure which has since been repeated here and in the United States.

Women planning donor insemination should not be alarmed by this. They do however need to know what the risks are and what precautions they should take. Basically you should make sure that the donor you are using has not been infected by HIV. At the moment this is determined by the HIV antibody test. Many of those who are antibody positive will still be carrying the virus and will be capable of passing it on if they donate semen. A negative result to the test *usually* means that the person is not infectious. Occasionally, however, the test produces false negatives. For this reason it is probably best not to use semen from men in high-risk groups, even if they have a negative antibody test. This includes sexually active gay or bisexual men, men who inject drugs and haemophiliacs. Another group who are high-risk for AIDS are men who have lived or worked in Central Africa, if sexual contact, or the sharing of needles or blood transfusion, has occurred.

Since the beginning of 1985, many centres offering artificial insemination have tested prospective donors for infection with HIV. The British Pregnancy Advisory Service, for instance, screens all its donors with the HIV antibody test.

You should insist on *frozen* sperm from a clinic that tests donors for HIV infection, preferably one that does not use sperm until the donor has been tested a second time a few months later. This is because in the early stages of infection the body does not produce antibodies to HIV. This means that if someone were tested shortly after having been infected the test would be negative, even though they may be carrying the virus. Retesting after a few months would solve this. In Australia, many clinics have a holding and retesting period of six months. This precludes the use of fresh semen.

If you are using a clinic be sure to ask if the donor's blood has been properly tested for HIV. Women doing self-insemination also need to be careful in choosing a donor. In the past gay men have often acted as donors. Now, with a high proportion of gay men thought to be infected with the virus, especially in the London area, gay men are being advised not to donate sperm and it would seem safest not to use them as donors. Men from other high-risk groups should also not act as donors, for similar reasons.

If you do decide to use a donor from a high-risk group you should make every attempt to find out how likely it is that they might have the virus. Apart from being asked detailed questions about their medical, social and sexual background, a prospective donor should have the HIV antibody test. For reasons I have already outlined, this would involve his taking the test twice, with a three-month gap. If both tests were negative, the sperm could be used *providing* that the donor had done nothing to put himself at risk of infection in the period between the first and second test. Otherwise there would be no knowing if the second negative result would, in a few months' time, become positive.

Some women who have used donors from high-risk groups, or who had artificial insemination before 1985 when screening for HIV was introduced, may be worried about the possibility of their developing AIDS. This is extremely unlikely. No cases of AIDS or HIV-related illness due to artificial insemination have so far been reported in this country or in the United States. It is possible to find out if you have been infected with HIV by having the antibody test. *However this is something you should think very carefully about before doing.* If you are extremely anxious or worried about the possibility of being infected with HIV then it may help to have the test. On the other hand if you do have the test you must be fully prepared to accept that it might turn out to be positive, a result which could have serious emotional and practical consequences. For women who are worried about whether they may be infected some of the pros and cons of taking the test are discussed in Chapter 7.

3 Lesbians and AIDS

What does AIDS have to do with lesbians? This is a question which you could be forgiven for asking. After all, very few lesbians are known to have got AIDS and, generally speaking, lesbians are considered to be a very low-risk group for AIDS and other sexually transmitted diseases.

Nevertheless, AIDS does affect lesbians in a number of ways. As health care workers and as workers in AIDS projects, lesbians are involved in the care of people with AIDS. Similarly, many lesbians have been affected by AIDS-related deaths or illnesses of gay men they know. Others may be anxious about going to mixed gay clubs or discos because they are afraid they might get AIDS. Lesbians are also affected by the strengthening of anti-gay feeling which the disease or, more accurately, its portrayal in the mass media has led to. In particular they may experience greater violence towards them because of AIDS. Also of concern to lesbians are the problems that AIDS raises for those considering artificial or self-insemination. Finally, lesbians are involved because, like other women, they too can get AIDS.

The main impact of AIDS on the lesbian community relates to the way in which AIDS has been seen, wrongly, as a 'gay disease' *and* the way in which lesbians have been categorised together with gay men. One consequence of this is that some lesbians have been refused as blood donors on the grounds that their 'homosexuality' puts them at risk. Nottingham Blood Transfusion Service, for example, refused last year to accept a woman's blood after she told them she was a lesbian. Shortly afterwards she received a letter stating the Service's policy of not accepting lesbian blood, because of the supposed risk of it being infected with HIV. In response to this Nottingham Lesbian Line campaigned and were successful in getting this policy changed on the grounds that lesbians are probably least at risk of AIDS.

Many lesbians have been insulted and threatened in connection with AIDS. Increased anti-gay hostility and discrimination as a result of the ignorance and hysteria which surround AIDS can affect lesbians in other ways. The reluctance of the courts to grant custody and, in some cases, access to lesbian mothers is well known. Behind these actions lies the assumption that lesbians do not make good mothers. This is very often based on a concern that children of a lesbian mother will grow up to be lesbian or gay themselves. This is a view which is not only discriminatory, in regarding being lesbian or gay as an undesirable outcome, but is also without foundation. More recently, a new objection to lesbian motherhood has emerged. In the United States a lesbian mother was denied visitation rights because of the judge's fear that she might give her children AIDS.

Historically there has been tension between the lesbian community and gay men. Nevertheless, many lesbians, especially in the United States, have played an important role in the development of AIDS organisations, fundraising and other forms of AIDS-related work. One example of lesbian involvement was the 'Our Brothers Need Blood' campaign in San Francisco. This, and similar campaigns in other American cities, was aimed at getting lesbians to donate blood in support of gay men. Women donated blood and credited their blood units to a special account, available to any person with AIDS in need of blood. The account was established to alleviate some of the costs incurred during a transfusion. In California, those who give blood are credited with blood units which can be used if they need a blood transfusion. Alternatively, you can credit your units to someone else. Those who don't donate blood, such as many gay men, have to pay for blood they receive. This is a situation that is made more difficult by the fact that many health insurance companies are reluctant to provide cover for gay men, especially if they are antibody positive, because they are a risk group for AIDS.

There are lesbians who, whilst they may sympathise with gay men over AIDS, feel it is important that they put their time and energy into issues of more direct relevance to women and, more especially, to other lesbians. Some lesbians feel angry that gay men, who have previously shown little interest or involvement in issues that concern women, now expect lesbians to support them. Such reactions are perhaps more likely amongst lesbians living in the UK than in America, as in the US there is a stronger tradition of lesbians and gay men working together in 'mixed' organisations.

A tension also exists between the lesbian and gay community and those who identify themselves as bisexual. Previously, lesbians have argued that bisexuals are sheltering under a label of comparative privilege. A woman who identifies herself as bisexual can have sexual relationships with other women without experiencing the same degree of social rejection that would be involved in a commitment to a lesbian identity. Now, with AIDS, some lesbians are also concerned that bisexual women may pass on AIDS to the lesbian community.

Who is at risk?

No one knows exactly how many lesbians have been diagnosed as having AIDS. This is not only because some women who have got AIDS may not want to 'admit' that they are lesbian. Both in the UK and the United States, women with AIDS are not classified according to their sexual preference. This is perhaps not surprising, given the lack of medical recognition of lesbian health issues in general. There is 'informal' reporting of lesbians with AIDS. In October 1985 the New York paper *The Village Voice* printed a story about a lesbian who had become infected with HIV, and subsequently developed AIDS, as a result of injecting drugs. Similarly, the Women's AIDS Network in San Francisco reports that of the few lesbians they know of in the United States who have AIDS, most fall into the category of injecting drug user.

Although specific figures are not available, the Centers for Disease Control, the organisation that is monitoring the AIDS epidemic in the United States, considers lesbians to be the lowest-risk group for AIDS. Consequently, most lesbians need worry very little about getting AIDS. Because of this we need to be very careful, in talking about lesbians and AIDS, not to create anxieties but rather to emphasise that most lesbians are not at risk. At the same time, lesbians should not see themselves as immune to the disease. *Anyone* can become infected with HIV given the relevant risk factors. Some lesbians may occasionally have sex with men who may be at risk. Some lesbians inject drugs.

Lesbians are at risk of being infected with HIV if they:

- Share needles or any other equipment for injecting drugs.
- Have had sex with men from high-risk groups over the last five years.
- Have used semen for artificial insemination from a donor who is infected with HIV.
- Have received blood transfusions or blood products with blood infected with HIV. (In the UK and in the United States this risk has largely been eliminated, since 1985, through the introduction of screening.)
- Have had sexual contact with women who have the virus.

It is lesbians who share needles or other equipment for mixing and injecting drugs who run the biggest risk of contracting HIV. Of the very few cases of AIDS among lesbians that have been reported in the United States, most have a history of injecting drug use. Lesbians are also at risk if they engage in unsafe sex with men from high-risk groups. As various studies have shown, there is no necessary association between regarding yourself as a lesbian and only having sex with women. Some lesbians do have sex with men. Nevertheless, many women do choose to have sexual relationships only with women. They, and other lesbians who decide that they want a child by artificial insemination, may be at risk if they use a donor from a high-risk group. In addition to the risk to themselves there is also the possibility, if they do become infected with HIV, that the virus could be passed on to any child they might have (see pages 47-51).

Since most clinics now screen would-be donors for HIV infection, this particularly applies to women who are carrying out insemination for themselves, without the help of an official donor organisation. That many lesbians prefer to do this is understandable. Though it is possible for lesbians to get AID through the NHS, the medical profession generally regards artificial insemination as a way of helping heterosexual couples conceive a child.

Insemination choices for lesbians have been limited because of AIDS. In the past, lesbians have often used gay men as donors. One of the advantages of this is that there would seem to be less likelihood of a gay man using a woman's lesbianism against her in a later dispute over the child. With the spread of AIDS, gay men are now being advised not to donate sperm. Although not all gay men are infected with HIV or have engaged in high-risk behaviours, a high proportion are thought to be affected. Studies of gay men attending STD clinics in the London area indicate that 20 per cent are infected with the virus. Lesbians planning self-insemination should therefore think very carefully about using gay men, or indeed any men from high-risk groups, as donors.

As a further safeguard it is important to get information about your donor's health and medical and sexual history. With the availability of the antibody test, many lesbians have also asked their donors to be tested. For the reasons which I have already outlined in the previous chapter, the antibody test should be done twice prior to insemination with a period of three to six months between tests. Your donor should practise safe sex between tests and should not engage in any other high-risk activities. If the second test is positive the donor's semen should not be used. If the test is negative then the semen will most probably be safe to use. There is however a slim chance that someone could have a negative test result and still be infected with the virus, especially if they are in a high-risk group. For this reason it may be advisable not to use a donor who is in a high-risk group, even if both tests are negative.

Research on the possible risk of infection with HIV from artificial/donor insemination is virtually non-existent. In San Francisco the Lesbian Insemination Project, a study of lesbians who have been inseminated since 1980, is the first study of its kind. (Since so many gay men in San Francisco are infected with the virus, and because many lesbians have used semen from gay men, questions about HIV infection have been critical for lesbians there.) In this study all the lesbians taking part were given the antibody test and, in addition, were asked to complete a questionnaire about their insemination history. According to Cheri Pies, co-ordinator of the study, many of the lesbians (at least half) used gay men as donors. Any women who are antibody positive may also have their lovers and children tested so that more can be learnt about how HIV may be transmitted from woman to woman or to children.

Thus far there have been no documented cases of a woman getting AIDS through sexual contact with another woman. Research is only just beginning on how well the virus lives in menstrual blood or vaginal and cervical fluids, and no one knows how or if women can sexually transmit HIV to other women. To ascertain this one would need to carry out studies of the female sexual partners of women who are antibody positive or who have AIDS. Needless to say, follow-up studies of the sexual partners of lesbians with HIV or AIDS are rare. In the Lesbian Insemination Project, none of the women who are sexual partners of women who have been inseminated, and are antibody positive, have yet developed any symptoms of AIDS.

Until more is known about the possibility of woman-to-woman transmission, lesbians are being advised to follow safe sex guidelines if they fall into one of the risk groups.

Safer sex

As lesbians, we rarely talk about what we do in bed. This silence around lesbian sex is an understandable reaction, given that it is the sexual aspects of being a lesbian that have tended to dominate how others see us. Another important reason is that sexual acts between women are very often interpreted as a 'turn on' for men, whether as pornography or not.

One of the consequences of not discussing our sex lives with other lesbians is that we often have to struggle alone, or with our lovers, in dealing with our sexual difficulties and worries. Breaking down the silence around lesbian sex is also important so that we can realistically assess what risks, if any, we are taking when it comes to sexually transmitted diseases such as AIDS.

It is important to re-emphasise, lest some lesbians become unnecessarily frightened or turned off sex, that lesbians are the lowest-risk group for AIDS within the sexually active population as a whole. Most lesbians need worry very little about getting AIDS, and will have no need to change their sexual behaviour. Those whose activities may place them at risk of HIV infection, however, do need to take precautions. (Safer sex for heterosexual women is discussed in the following chapter.)

Concern about AIDS doesn't mean that you can't have sex. Rather, it means that you may have to change the type of sexual practices you enjoy, in situations where either you or your lover may be at risk. Because they are likely to have more control over their sexuality, this may be easier for lesbians than for women having sexual relationships with men. In a study at the AIDS Foundation in San Francisco, women were interviewed who were having sexual contact with high-risk men. The majority said that they were afraid of bringing up the issue of safe sex for fear of being rejected, or of the men being unreceptive. Similarly, because the act of 'penetration' does not have the same meaning or significance for lesbian lovemaking as it does for heterosexual sex, a woman's female lover is less likely to regard 'safe sex' as dull or unexciting sex.

There are many ways in which women enjoy making love with one another. These include kissing on the mouth, kissing or caressing other parts of the body, touching or licking the clitoris and labia, stimulation of the breasts and nipples and rubbing against each other. Some women also like their vaginas to be touched at some point during lovemaking. However, contrary to popular belief, and male pornography, the use of dildos is relatively rare.

In recent years sado-masochistic (s/m) and other practices such as 'fist-fucking' have been the subject of heated controversy among lesbians. This is an important debate which deserves further discussion. Unfortunately, within the context of this book there is not the space to do justice to the arguments about why many lesbians object to such practices.

What activities put lesbians at risk for HIV infection? Most importantly, you should avoid sex which involves contact with body fluids. The body fluids you need to be concerned about are semen, blood (including menstrual blood), vaginal secretions, urine, faeces and breast milk. Although HIV has been found in saliva, there is no evidence that it can be transmitted this way.

In order for infection to occur the virus must be transmitted into the bloodstream. Certain sexual practices and blood transfusion through shared needles allow that to happen. Therefore, if you believe that you or your partner may be infected with the virus, or you are not sure, you should avoid body fluids coming into contact with your mouth, rectum, vagina or any break in the skin through which the virus might gain entrance to the bloodstream.

Low-risk lesbian sex

There is little or no need to worry about becoming infected through:

- Hugging or massaging each other.
- Touching your own genitals.
- Kissing. There is no evidence of HIV having been transmitted solely through exposure to saliva. The only time when kissing might spread the virus would be through 'wet kissing', in which large amounts of saliva are passed. Provided neither partner has open cuts or sores of the mouth, lips or tongue, kissing probably represents little or no risk.
- Body-to-body rubbing.
- Body kissing.
- Sharing sexual fantasies.
- Using vibrators, or other sex toys, *providing* that they are not shared or are cleaned and dried thoroughly between each partner's use.
- Activities that do not involve the exchange of body fluids.

Medium-risk lesbian sex

- Oral sex. Oral sex, or cunnilingus, is where one woman stimulates her lover's genitals with her mouth or tongue. Oral sex carries some risk because there is a chance that the virus may be transmitted through vaginal fluids. It has been suggested that cunnilingus may be less risky if it is done using a latex or rubber barrier that prevents the exchange of fluids between the tongue and the vulva. However, no research has been done on whether or not such barriers provide protection against HIV infection, and many people may find them awkward to use.
- Hand/finger-to-genital contact. This includes activities such as 'mutual masturbation' and vaginal or anal 'penetration' with fingers. If you have cuts, scratches or sores on your fingers or hands, wearing surgical rubber gloves will reduce the risk of coming into contact with the virus.
- External urine contact ('watersports').
- Oral-anal contact (rimming) *with* a barrier.

Higher-risk lesbian sex

- Unprotected cunnilingus/oral sex, especially during menstruation since menstrual blood may contain the virus.
- Unprotected hand-vagina or hand-anal contact, especially if you have cuts, scratches or sores on your hands or fingers.
- Unprotected oral-anal contact.
- Urine or faeces in the mouth or vagina.
- Sharing sex toys, such as vibrators, that have come into contact with body fluids could be risky, as they could carry the infection from one person to another.
- Fisting (hand in rectum/vagina). Because the walls of

the rectum can be easily injured during 'fisting' the inserting partner's fingers or hand may be exposed to her partner's blood. Any practice that breaks the skin or draws blood, either inside the vagina or anus or on the skin, will increase the risk of getting the virus.

- Related to this, any type of blood contact, including menstrual blood, is unsafe.

Lesbians who inject drugs are also at risk for AIDS and should not, *under any circumstances*, share needles or other equipment for mixing and injecting drugs. The risks associated with injecting drug use and how to reduce them by coming off or changing the way you use drugs are discussed on pages 26-30.

A worry some lesbians may have, despite the fact so very few lesbians have got AIDS, is how do I know if my new lover is at risk? The simple answer is to ask her. If you have a new sexual partner find out about her history and share your own. Do either of you, for instance, have a history of injecting drugs or having sex with men from high-risk groups? Telling other lesbians that you have slept with men, or admitting that you inject drugs, can be a difficult thing to do. However, it is vital if you think you may be at risk that you let your partner(s) know. By talking it will be possible to realistically assess whether, like most lesbians, you are not at risk of either getting or passing on HIV or, alternatively, you need to follow safe sex guidelines.

If you have sex with men you should make every effort to find out if they are at risk of being infected with HIV and, if they are, follow the safe sex guidelines described in the following chapter. Remember, having sex with another woman carries *much* less risk of AIDS, and other sexually transmitted diseases, than heterosexual intercourse.

Lesbians with AIDS

Lesbians who have AIDS may experience special problems given that the health care system is designed for
and administered by a predominantly heterosexual population. Staff may hold negative attitudes about lesbianism,
making it difficult for lesbians to feel comfortable,
especially in expressing physical affection towards their
women friends and lovers. Similarly, some hospital
regulations may discriminate against lesbians. Visiting
rules, for example, may specify 'immediate family only'.
Whilst you can put down who you like as next-of-kin, not
all lesbians may be aware of this. This could cause a great
deal of distress if hospital staff do not recognise that
lesbians may regard their lovers as next-of-kin.

This may also apply when a woman dies from AIDS.
The feelings one has when one's lover dies are no less
painful for lesbians than for anyone else. What is
different, often, is the context in which the process of
mourning takes place. Lesbian relationships are not
socially recognised or accepted in the same way that
heterosexual or family relationships are. As a consequence of this a lesbian may not be invited to her lover's
funeral and, if no will was made, may have to face the
ordeal of her dead lover's family sharing out savings or
possessions. This is one reason why it is important to
make a will.

Clearly the process of mourning will be much more
difficult for women who are isolated and have no one to
talk to about how they feel. Even those lesbians who have
the support of others may experience this to some degree
if, for example, they have not come out at work or to their
family. The gay bereavement project is a 24-hour service
providing practical and emotional support for lesbians
and gay men whose lovers have died. They can also give
advice about making wills and funeral arrangements.
They can be contacted through London Lesbian and Gay

Switchboard, whose number is listed at the end of the book.

One of the problems in telling others that you are a lesbian is the hostile and violent reactions that this can evoke. It can also mean having to deal with rejection. For example, one of the problems lesbians have in coming out to parents is that parents may assume, wrongly, that this is somehow their 'fault'. Typically this leads to the woman being blamed by her parents, who at the same time feel guilty for causing what they do not want to accept in their daughter. For those women who may be forced to come out as a lesbian while they are seriously ill, encountering such reactions will be especially stressful.

4 Safer sex

Anyone who is sexually active can get AIDS through sexual contact. The only exception is the couple who have *both* had sex only with each other for at least five years, and have not used shared needles to inject drugs, had transfusions, or used other blood products. All sexually active women, particularly those whose partners are in a high-risk group or who are unsure of the sexual background of their partners, need to know about ways of reducing the risk of contracting the virus which can lead to AIDS.

Apart from access to information about AIDS, the degree of control women have in sexual relationships with men will seriously affect how able they are to reduce their risk of HIV infection. For instance, a man can choose to protect himself by wearing a condom, but a woman has to ask a man to agree to this.

Communication is vital to safe sex. It is important that you say what you want, and negotiate what you can do together. Given the nature of male-female relationships, many women will find this a difficult thing to do. They may not feel able to talk about sex with their male partner, especially at the start of a sexual relationship, perhaps because they would feel too embarrassed or are afraid of how he would react. There may also be economic or cultural reasons why a woman may not feel that she has much say over what happens in bed. Within some marriages sex may be almost a bargain, part of what a husband expects of a wife in return for supporting her.

Although there is no reason to believe that men are incapable of making changes in their sexual behaviour, many men may be reluctant to do so. The reasons for this are complex and relate to the meanings attached to sex. As part of the social construction of male sexuality, many men come to believe that sex is both more important and more uncontrollable for them than it is for women, that men and not women should take the sexual initiative and that what counts as having sex is penetration of the vagina by the penis. In addition to this, having sex, but more especially having sexual intercourse, is seen as a central aspect of being masculine and male. One reason therefore why men, both heterosexual and gay, may be unwilling to alter their sexual behaviour in the light of AIDS is that such changes would represent a threat to their identity. Another possible reason is that they do not see safe sex as erotic. While some men may be willing to agree that satisfying sex need not imply intercourse, others will not. For them safe sex may seem dull or uninteresting sex, which would impose too many restrictions on their sexual pleasure. Recognising this, many of the risk reduction guidelines make a point of emphasising that safe sex can be fun, exciting and satisfying. (In the United States workshops on eroticising safe sex, and safe sex pornography and erotica, are examples of attempts being made to change sexual attitudes and behaviour among men.)

Because of the different meanings attached to female sexuality, women are likely to need less convincing of this than men. Sexual surveys show that, generally speaking, women are more dissatisfied with their sex lives than are men and that, very often, their dissatisfaction is related to sex being defined primarily as intercourse. The fact that AIDS forces us to question many of the assumptions we hold about sex may, therefore, in some ways be regarded as positive.

This is not to ignore the fact that for some women AIDS has meant sexual difficulties. If they or their partner has AIDS, is antibody positive or thinks they may be infected with the virus, anxieties about the consequences of having sex may lead to a loss of sexual desire. Some women may also be worried and fearful about sex because they are unsure about whether their partner may have had sex with someone who might be at risk, and not told them. Such fears will be even greater for women whose partners expect and, in some cases, force them to have risky sex.

How women feel about safer sex will also depend on what sex, and certain sexual practices in particular, means to them. To what extent is sex an important part of their lives and how they see themselves? What kinds of sex do they enjoy most? How many different partners have they had over the past year? The difficulties women may have in making changes in their sexual behaviour are likely to depend on the answers to these and similar sorts of questions. For example, some women may experience difficulties in adapting to risk reduction guidelines because they feel frustrated at the thought of having to have fewer sexual partners. Whilst this is seen as something that men are likely to experience, the assumption that women both want and find it easy to be monogamous has meant little thought has been given to how women might feel about this. Equally, the assumption that sex isn't as important to women may result in AIDS-related sexual difficulties and fears in women being ignored.

How can a woman reduce her risk of AIDS?

There are several ways in which you can reduce your risk of becoming infected with HIV and, possibly, developing AIDS. Basically speaking it is important that you avoid having sex which involves an exchange of body fluids with men or women who may be at risk for HIV infection, their sexual partners, or with people who have AIDS or HIV-related disease.

If you already have AIDS, are antibody positive or think you might be infected with the virus, you should *always* follow risk reduction guidelines. Some people may feel that if they have already been infected with HIV they have nothing to lose by continuing to engage in unsafe sex. However, even though they may not have AIDS, they may be infectious to others and those persons may get AIDS. In addition to this, some doctors believe that repeated exposure to the virus may increase the likelihood of a person developing AIDS. By following risk reduction guidelines a woman may therefore reduce the risk to herself of getting AIDS, even though she is already infected with HIV.

The risk of acquiring any sexually transmitted disease rises with the number of different sexual partners you have. Similarly, with AIDS the more people you have sex with the more likely it is that at least one of them will be infected with the virus that causes it. This is especially true if you have sex with people from high-risk groups. One way of reducing the risk of catching the virus therefore is to be more selective about who you have sex with. (However, being monogamous is no protection against AIDS if your partner is already infected with HIV.) Know your sexual partner, his state of health, his lifestyle and his sexual habits. Avoid having sex with men you know little or nothing about. Talk to any potential sexual partner and ascertain whether he is at risk for AIDS *before* you make love. (Likewise make your own risk status known to him.) Ask him if you are the only sexual partner he has? Does he have sex with other men, even occasionally? Does he ever inject drugs and share needles with other users?

One of the difficulties for women in doing this, apart from any embarrassment which they may feel, is that men may not answer their questions truthfully. When

Below is a list of different ways of having sex. Some of the ways are described as low-risk. These are activities which are believed to carry little or no risk of the virus being passed from one person to another. Others are marked medium-risk because it is thought that they carry a risk of transmitting the virus, although not as much risk as the types of sex listed as high-risk.

Low-risk
- Massage.
- Hugging.
- Kissing.
- Body-to-body rubbing.
- Sex toys, providing they are not shared.
- Body kissing.
- Mutual masturbation.
- Sharing sexual fantasies.
- Any sexual activities that do not involve the exchange of body fluids.

Medium-risk
- Oral sex by a man to a woman (or woman to woman). Using a barrier may reduce the risk.
- Hand/finger-to-genital contact without a latex or rubber glove (e.g. vaginal or anal penetration with fingers).
- Vaginal intercourse with a condom.
- Anal intercourse with a condom.
- Oral sex by a woman to a man (fellatio) using a condom.

High-risk
- Vaginal intercourse, without a condom.
- Anal intercourse (using a *strong* condom and plenty of water-based lubricant reduces the risk).
- Semen, urine or faeces in the mouth or vagina.
- Fisting (hand in rectum/vagina).
- Sharing sex toys.
- Rimming (oral-anal contact).
- Oral sex by a woman to a man (fellatio) without using a condom.
- Any type of blood contact (including menstrual blood).

you are not sure if a man may be infected with HIV either don't have sex with him or follow risk reduction (safe sex) guidelines, unless you want to run the risk of becoming infected yourself. Avoid using alcohol and drugs when you have sex. They may impair your judgment, affecting decisions about who you have sex with and what kind of sex you have.

Some ways of having sex are more likely to transmit the virus than others. For transmission to occur, body fluids containing HIV must enter a woman's body through her vagina, rectum, mouth or breaks in the skin. The exchange of blood and semen carries the highest risk of infection, but other body fluids and products, such as urine and faeces, may also transmit the virus. Activities that do not involve the exchange or passing of any body fluids between partners are believed to be safe.

Having said this, there is disagreement over what may or may not be safe sex. This is hardly surprising given that there is so much that is still not known about HIV and how it is transmitted. In the light of this some prefer to use the term *safer* sex or risk reduction.

No one can be certain about what is totally safe. Only you can decide what is a reasonable amount of risk. Hopefully, the following guidelines will help you to make informed choices. Though it includes information of relevance to all women, this section is primarily aimed at women in heterosexual relationships. Information on safer sex for lesbians is contained in the previous chapter.

Anal sex

Studies have shown that anal sex is the main way in which HIV is sexually transmitted among men. Women can also catch HIV through anal as well as vaginal intercourse.

The walls of the rectum are designed to absorb fluids readily and are very thin. They can easily be damaged during anal intercourse, allowing the virus to enter the bloodstream, carried either by semen or by blood from an injury to the penis. Even if there is no tissue damage, it may be possible for semen carrying HIV to get into the bloodstream during anal intercourse.

By far the safest solution is to avoid anal sex. However if, despite the risks, you are having anal sex you should insist that your partner wears a condom. Although it is not known how effective they are in real-life situations, studies have shown that condoms can prevent the transmission of HIV in the laboratory. For this reason most researchers believe that, when used properly, condoms may reduce the risk of contracting HIV during vaginal and anal intercourse.

Since condoms can fall off or tear during sex, a further measure of protection is for the man to withdraw his penis before he ejaculates. The major causes of condoms breaking are air inside the condom, not enough lubrication, old or faulty condoms, or the use of oil-based lubricants.

Apart from helping to prevent the condom from ripping, the use of a lubricant during anal sex will also help to reduce friction and possible damage to the rectal walls. If you use a lubricant you should make sure it is a water-based lubricant like KY Jelly or Duragel. You should not use Vaseline or any oil-based lubricant, as they dissolve the rubber.

There is some evidence that nonoxynol-9, a chemical agent which is found in most spermicides and some lubricants, may afford some protection against HIV infection. Although it is not usual, some women are allergic to nonoxynol-9. You should therefore first test any product containing nonoxynol-9 on the inside of your wrist before using it for sex. If you do get an allergic reaction try using a different brand.

Another way of reducing the risk, and the worry, associated with the condom breaking is to use a *strong* condom. Redstripe or Prophyltex is supposed to be thicker and stronger than other condoms currently on the market. It also contains the spermicide nonoxynol-9. This type of condom can be got from STD clinics or by mail order from FTC, Ladbroke Grove, London W11 3BG or Clovelink & Patmark Chemists, Praed St, London W2.

Other forms of anal sex, besides anal intercourse, are equally dangerous. Putting vibrators or other sex toys into the rectum could be risky as they could pass the virus from one person to another if they are shared. 'Fisting', inserting the entire hand into the rectum and balling it into a fist, is likely to cause tears in the walls of the rectum. Apart from the risk of infection with HIV through the exchange of blood, this can lead to a number of other very serious, potentially fatal injuries and infections, such as peritonitis. If, despite these risks, you do this you or your partner should always use a surgical glove. Similarly, if you have cuts or scratches on your fingers wearing a disposable rubber glove will reduce the risk of becoming infected with HIV during anal penetration with fingers. Throw the glove away afterwards. Disposable rubber gloves can be bought in most chemists.

Although there is no evidence so far of HIV being transmitted through faeces, any sexual practice which involves contact with faeces is regarded as high-risk, as it may contain blood. This includes oral-anal contact, also known as analingus or 'rimming'. Apart from the possibility of contracting HIV, oral contact with faeces may lead to a number of serious infectious diseases, such as hepatitis. Whilst it is safest to avoid these activities, using a barrier that prevents the exchange of fluids between the tongue and the anus *may* reduce the risk of HIV transmission if you do have oral-anal sex. 'Rubber dams', or latex barriers, which are a thin piece of latex about the same thickness as a disposable rubber glove, can be used for this. However it is important to remember that at this time it is not known to what extent these provide protection against HIV infection.

Vaginal intercourse

While anal sex may be a particularly easy way for a woman to contract the virus, vaginal intercourse also carries a high degree of risk for infection with HIV. HIV can be transmitted in semen entering the vagina. The virus might get into the bloodstream through ulcerations or erosions of the cervix or, possibly, through the vaginal walls. Though much thicker than the rectum, the walls of the vagina contain many blood vessels which become swollen with blood during sexual arousal. Cuts or sores on a woman's genitals may also allow the virus to enter her bloodstream, carried either by semen or by blood from the man's penis.

Many researchers believe that the risk of the virus being transmitted from a man to a woman during sexual intercourse is greater than the other way around. Studies both of gay men and female partners of men who inject drugs, for instance, suggest that it is the person *receiving* semen who is at greater risk of infection during intercourse. Nevertheless, sexual transmission of HIV from women to men can occur. The vaginal secretions of infected women may contain the virus, though it is thought that menstrual blood from women carrying the virus probably holds a greater risk of infection. As with male-female transmission, the virus may be passed more easily from a woman to a man if there are cuts or abrasions on the penis which would allow the virus more direct access to the bloodstream.

One way of eliminating this risk is not to have intercourse. Because this demands the co-operation of men, it may be difficult to achieve in practice. It's no good a woman wanting to make love without having intercourse if the man she is having sex with won't agree.

If you do have intercourse, your male partner should always use a condom. Condoms cannot provide absolute assurance since they can come off, or break, but most researchers believe that used properly they may offer some degree of protection from HIV both to the woman and her male partner. Many studies have shown them to be effective in preventing other sexually transmitted diseases such as gonorrhea, syphilis and herpes.

Condoms should be used with a spermicide containing nonoxynol-9. A further measure of protection is for the man to withdraw before ejaculation, since the condom may break. If you use a lubricant it should be water-soluble, such as KY. The reasons for this have already been discussed.

Condoms are readily available, relatively inexpensive, and, with practice, are easy to use. (The Family Planning Association provides free condoms for contraceptive use but not disease prevention.) They have no adverse side-effects and when used in conjunction with a spermicide are an effective means of birth control. Their serious disadvantage for women is that it is necessary to get men to agree to use them. While this will not be a problem for all women, some men don't like and may refuse to wear a condom and, in some cases, may force a woman to engage in unprotected intercourse.

Apart from the risk of infection with HIV, vaginal intercourse can result in pregnancy. As I have discussed earlier, pregnancy in antibody positive women may lead to the virus being passed on to the child as well as, possibly, increasing their own chances of developing AIDS. If you or your partner are in a high-risk group, or if either of you have been diagnosed as having HIV, then you should consider deferring pregnancy. This is discussed in more detail in Chapter 2. While alternative forms of birth control to the condom, such as the pill or an IUD, may be effective in preventing pregnancy, they will not reduce your risk of becoming infected with HIV. Therefore, you should *always* use a condom during vaginal intercourse, irrespective of whether or not you are already using some other method of contraception.

Other forms of vaginal sex also carry a risk. Inserting

fingers or a hand into a woman's vagina – 'fisting' – may involve the exchange of blood. Wearing a surgical rubber glove, especially if the person has cuts or scratches on their hand or fingers, may reduce this risk. Apart from semen and blood, you should also not allow urine or faeces to come into contact with your vagina. Sharing sex toys that have come into contact with bodily fluids should be avoided.

Oral sex

Oral sex is where one partner stimulates the other's genitals with their mouth or tongue. When a woman (or man) does this to a man it is called fellatio. The term used when a man (or woman) does this to a woman is cunnilingus.

Whether the virus can be transmitted orally, either by oral-genital or oral-anal contact, is not clear. However, until more is known about HIV and how it is transmitted, oral sex should be considered to carry some degree of risk. In fellatio this is because the virus could pass from the man's semen into the woman's body. The best way to avoid this is not having your partner ejaculate in your mouth. Even if you do not swallow his semen there may be some risk of infection if there are cuts or sores in and around your mouth and gums that would allow the virus to enter the bloodstream. Apart from the risk from infected semen, there is also the risk of being exposed to blood infected with HIV if your partner has any small cuts or abrasions on his penis. Withdrawing his penis before ejaculation does not totally avoid the risk from semen, since many men produce some secretion from the penis prior to ejaculation.

For men fellatio probably carries little or no risk of infection. Although the virus has been isolated in saliva, the exchange of saliva is generally thought to be low-risk for HIV infection. (Men who carry out fellatio for their male partners obviously run the same risks as women who do this.)

If you carry out oral sex for a man he should wear a condom to reduce the risk of infection to you. However, since a condom can break, he should withdraw before ejaculation as a further measure of protection. Once again, the question of how much control women have within sexual relationships with men is a critical one.

Cunnilingus is also thought to carry some degree of risk. Unless it contains blood the risk of HIV being transmitted through saliva is generally thought to be low. If there are no cuts or sores on a woman's genital area it is therefore unlikely that she will become infected by her partner during oral sex. The main risk is to the man (or woman) doing this to her. The cervical and vaginal secretions of women infected with HIV may contain the virus. HIV is also likely to be present in a woman's menstrual blood. Therefore, if the man (or woman) carrying out oral sex has bleeding gums, mouth ulcers or any breaks in the skin in or around the mouth, the virus may be able to get into the bloodstream.

As the exchange of blood (and semen) is thought to carry a higher risk for infection with HIV than cervical and vaginal fluids, you should especially avoid having oral sex during a period. Some researchers have suggested that using a thin rubber barrier, that would prevent the exchange of fluids between the tongue and the vulva, *may* reduce the risk of infection with HIV. However at present no studies have been done on whether or not 'rubber dams' or latex barriers can prevent transmission of HIV.

Kissing

The only time when kissing might spread the virus would be through French ('wet') kissing, where large amounts of saliva are exchanged. Even then, the risk is likely to be low unless the saliva contains blood. While the virus has been found in saliva, there are no reports of people being infected by this form of transmission. Providing there are no breaks in the skin that could result in your being exposed to their blood, kissing your partner's body also carries little risk of acquiring HIV.

Masturbation

'Mutual masturbation' is where both partners stimulate the other's genitals with their hands. Whether it is done mutually, or only involves one person touching another, there is a very low risk of transmitting HIV through hand-to-genital contact. If you masturbate your male partner and have cuts, scratches or sores on your fingers and hands, wearing surgical rubber gloves will reduce the risk of your coming into contact with semen containing the virus. Similarly, wearing surgical gloves will reduce the risk of exposure to blood and cervical and vaginal fluids for men (and women) who stimulate a woman's genitals with their hands.

Activities such as biting or scratching, that may result in your blood coming into contact with an infected partner's blood or semen, carry some degree of risk. Sharing sex toys such as vibrators could also result in the virus being transmitted from one person to another. Any kind of sex which involves contact with urine or faeces is also considered to be associated with the risk of infection.

Safe sex

In outlining risk reduction guidelines it is important to include things that people can do, as well as things that are best avoided.

Any sexual activity that does *not* involve the exchange or passing of body fluids between partners is of low or no risk (assuming that the uninfected partner does not have any open cuts, grazes, sores, etc.). Hugging, rubbing against each other's bodies, cuddling, stroking and massaging do not involve the exchange of body fluids and are safe. Sharing sexual fantasies is also safe. It is also considered safe for a man to ejaculate semen on to his partner's body, providing there are no cuts or breaks in the skin. Using vibrators or other sex toys carries no risk, providing that they are not shared or are cleaned and dried *thoroughly* between each partner's use.

Safe sex is not just about AIDS. Safe sex won't get you pregnant. Safe sex won't transmit any sexually transmitted disease. Far from being a restrictive influence, safe sex may encourage new ways of making love which broaden our enjoyment of sex.

5 Living with AIDS

Most of what has been written about what it's like to have AIDS has been about gay men. There has been very little analysis of the experience of women who have AIDS or who are antibody positive.

This is a serious omission. The problems AIDS creates for women are not necessarily the same as those for men – gay or otherwise. For instance, women's access to health care, the support systems available to them, their ability to make changes in their sex life and their reactions to physical decline and disfigurement are likely to be different to men's. In addition there are specific problems which AIDS creates for women, such as in pregnancy.

Whilst it is important to discover how women feel, this will not be easy. Most women with AIDS or who are antibody positive are reluctant to be interviewed. This is understandable. AIDS is a stigmatising illness. At present, very few women in this country have AIDS which makes them all the more easily identifiable.

Finding out

Margaret is in her early thirties. Two years ago she found out that she was antibody positive. She has never abused drugs and is not in any other risk group other than that her husband has haemophilia and unknowingly passed the virus on to her.

However much they are expecting it, for most people the news that they have AIDS or are antibody positive comes as a tremendous shock. This is how Margaret felt:

'As soon as we sat in the doctor's office and he told us I thought, Oh God, what's hit us! I thought someone had hit me over the head with a hammer. I was just confused. I didn't know what to do. I didn't know what to expect.'

Understandably, it can be difficult to take in information about the nature of the disease, how it is transmitted, what the possible implications of infection may be and so forth, whilst being in this kind of state. Nevertheless, there are a number of issues which women with HIV infection, or AIDS, need to know about soon after diagnosis.

First, it is important they understand that they will most likely be infectious, even if they do not have any symptoms of infection themselves. Women who are aware of this may initially worry a great deal about the risk they pose to others. Very often, this is due to a misunderstanding of how HIV is transmitted. It is essential that women with AIDS, or who are antibody positive, have access to *accurate* information about how the virus is passed on and the steps that they can take to reduce the risk of this happening. Even then they may need reassurance. Margaret admits to being worried about giving the virus to others, despite the fact that she knows nothing she does is likely to put them at risk. 'I am terrified in case we give it to someone else. I know we couldn't really, but it's just the thought. It's silly to worry but I do.'

Some of the precautions that women who are antibody positive or have AIDS should take are listed on page 84.

In addition to information about how they can reduce the risk of passing the virus on to others, it is also important for women with AIDS or HIV to know how they can reduce their own chances of getting ill. The list on page 85 includes suggestions for improving – or maintaining – one's health. Some researchers believe that such measures may be helpful in the treatment of AIDS, as well as reducing the risk of those who are infected with HIV going on to get the disease. While there is no evidence for this, many people report feeling better as a result of making healthy changes in their diet and way of life.

It can be difficult to get across to someone that being infected with HIV does not necessarily mean they will get AIDS. Nevertheless, it is important that women with the virus understand this. It is also important that they know what the symptoms of AIDS and related illness are so that they can monitor their own health and, if necessary, seek treatment quickly.

If I have AIDS or am antibody positive what precautions should I take?

- Do not give blood or carry an organ donor card.
- If you have sex with someone follow the risk reduction guidelines described in Chapter 4 and, for lesbians, Chapter 3.
- Do not share needles or other equipment for injecting drugs.
- Avoid becoming pregnant.
- Do not breastfeed your child.
- Cover any cuts or grazes with a waterproof plaster.
- Avoid sharing toothbrushes or razors, or anything likely to be contaminated with blood.
- Clean up any spilt blood or other body fluids immediately. Wash the surface down with household bleach diluted with ten parts of water.
- Dirty clothes, linen, towels, etc. should be washed in the hot wash cycle of an ordinary washing machine.
- Used sanitary towels and tampons should be flushed down the toilet, burnt or put into a sealed plastic bag and disposed of.

What should I do to protect my own health if I am antibody positive or have AIDS?

- Eat a properly balanced diet and, if you eat meat, make sure it is well cooked.
- Cut down or cut out drugs which may damage your immune system.
- Reduce the amount of stress in your life.
- Get enough rest and sleep.
- Practise 'safer sex' to avoid acquiring sexually transmitted diseases, which may worsen your immune status.
- Wash your hands after handling pets and avoid contact with their wastes.
- Avoid going to places where the sanitary conditions are poor and where there is a high risk of your developing infections. Normal standards of hygiene will be enough to protect you from household germs. Staying away from pubs, restaurants, cinemas, etc. is unnecessary.
- Do not accept any kind of vaccination unless your doctor knows that you are immune-deficient. While there is no risk from vaccines which contain killed virus, many vaccines have living – but altered – viruses which might cause problems for someone with immune deficiency.

Apart from access to basic information, women should also have the opportunity to discuss how they feel. A woman who is diagnosed as having AIDS or HIV has many issues which she will need to think about and come to terms with. Among these issues are treatment options, reactions by employers, family and friends, risk reduction, stigma and AIDS discrimination, feeling depressed and anxious, the physical effects of her condition, and dependency and finding support. In the following sections some of these are discussed in more detail.

AIDS discrimination

Women with AIDS or HIV infection can face many problems. Some of these may be due to the way in which people who have AIDS or are antibody positive are treated. AIDS is a severely stigmatising illness. There are stories of nurses refusing to change bedpans, feed, wash or even talk to someone in their care who has AIDS. In some cases people have been evicted from their homes, or have lost their job, once it became known that they were infected with HIV or had AIDS. Insurance companies are unwilling to provide life cover. There are reports of people being abandoned by their friends, relatives and lovers, of children being excluded from schools and of doctors refusing medical care.

Whatever form it takes, AIDS discrimination will be extremely distressing for those who have the disease or are antibody positive. Some may respond angrily. Others, terrified of being found out, may become very anxious and withdrawn.

Isolation

Women with AIDS or HIV infection are often socially isolated. This may be because of the way people who are misinformed about AIDS and how it is spread react to them: with fear and avoidance. For many, such a response generates a feeling of being 'dirty' or 'unclean' and they may choose not to discuss their diagnosis with others for fear of how they will react.

The issue of who to tell is one that Margaret has had to deal with. Apart from hospital staff, only her close family know that both she and her husband are antibody positive. The decision not to tell friends or neighbours has affected their social life.

'We stopped going out for months, just in case someone we met knew and they said anything. I didn't even think my mother should have known. I just didn't feel as if I trusted anyone to know, in case they mentioned it. What worries me about other people knowing is that they will treat me or my husband differently. I would have fears of them not speaking, or just passing in the street, or not coming anywhere near the house.'

There are other reasons, besides the fear that her friends will desert her, why a woman who is antibody positive or has AIDS may become socially withdrawn. She may be worried about infecting others. She may also be concerned about the risk others present to her, in terms of catching germs and diseases. A woman's social life will also be affected by the physical effects of her diagnosis. Women with AIDS or ARC (AIDS-related complex) may be too ill, or too easily tired, to be able to go out or socialise often.

Another reason why someone with AIDS may not mix socially is because they feel too upset or embarrassed about their physical appearance. Apart from weight loss, a person with AIDS may have disfiguring lesions on the face as well as other parts of the body. Those who undergo chemotherapy may also lose their hair. The impact of feeling unattractive on a person's self-esteem will vary. However given that – far more than men – women are frequently judged in terms of how they look, such changes may be particularly stressful for women.

Whatever the reasons for social isolation, it is important that women who have HIV infection, or AIDS, have someone to talk to. Often it is practical problems which a woman feels she needs to discuss, as well as her fears and anxieties. A lover, friend or relative may be able to provide this. Alternatively, it may be helpful to join a self-help group.

Meeting someone who is going through a similar experience to herself is something Margaret feels she would like to do.

'I feel very isolated and alone knowing that I don't know anyone in the same boat as me. They probably couldn't tell me anything I didn't already know, but I think it would just be nice to meet someone like me, because I would know what they'd be going through. I know there must be other women, but as far as I'm concerned I'm the only one. I just feel dead lonely.'

Another advantage in joining a support group for women in a similar situation to oneself is that it offers the opportunity of meeting others without the fear of being rejected or ostracised.

Few support groups for women with AIDS or who are antibody positive exist at present, though a number of voluntary organisations do offer advice and support to women. In the London area, the Terrence Higgins Trust can put you in touch with other women in the same position as yourself or arrange for someone to visit you. Both this and a number of other organisations offering help are listed on pages 137-41.

Anxiety

Most people when they discover they have AIDS feel shocked and disorientated. They may refuse to accept the diagnosis and become angry. Alternatively, they may react by blaming themselves for having the disease and feel depressed. Almost everyone feels anxious and scared.

Anxiety is something we all experience at different times in our lives. In this context, however, the anxiety felt is likely to be far more severe and longer-lasting. This is understandable. A diagnosis of AIDS is very frightening. It is a fatal disease for which there is currently no known cure.

Knowing that she may develop AIDS is something Margaret feels anxious about. Whereas she rarely worried about her health before being told she was HIV positive, she now has to confront the possibility that both she and her husband could become ill or even die.

'I worry about the future. Well, I've always been scared of dying anyway, always. When I lie there and I think my life could be cut short . . . I'm terrified if anything happens to me. For instance, I'm scared now if I get a cold, I make sure I get it seen to straight away. I'm always at the doctor's. I worry about my husband as well. If he's not well I think has he got it? If something happened through haemophilia I could come to terms with that: it's dying of AIDS I worry about. That's very upsetting. I cry about that a lot.'

The fact that AIDS occurs primarily in young adults makes the prospect of death even more difficult to accept. For many, however, the fear of death is not as great as the fear of dying a slow and painful death, isolated from people they know and care about.

Being rejected by family and friends is something that women with AIDS and HIV infection are likely to be afraid of. In addition, those already in a relationship may worry about how their lover will cope with the diagnosis and the issues it raises. In particular, they may be anxious about how the sexual implications will affect their relationship, and whether their lover will leave them for someone else. Those who work may also be frightened that they will lose their job if their employer finds out about their condition.

There is still a great deal that is not known or understood about AIDS. In view of this it is easy to see how women who have the disease, or have been diagnosed as positive on the HIV antibody test, may feel anxious for other reasons. For those with AIDS there is the uncertainty about how the disease will progress, the risks they pose to others, the effects of medical treatment and the possibility of a cure being developed. For those who have ARC, PGL (persistent generalised lymphadenopathy; see Glossary) or who are antibody positive, there is the uncertainty of whether they will go on to develop AIDS.

For many this is a constant source of anxiety, and they may be able to think of little else but the prospect of developing AIDS and what the consequences of this would be. Often this means going over and over the same thoughts. For instance, they may be worried that perhaps they have given the virus to someone else already. Or they may be consumed by thoughts of death and dying and watch themselves daily for symptoms. In some cases the anxiety produced by such thoughts is so great that this develops into an obsession. The person feels compelled to check their body for signs of illness and may spend many hours each day doing this. In this context, for all of the tragedy, bitterness and anger that a diagnosis of AIDS can bring, there may also be a kind of relief from the anxiety and uncertainty of not knowing whether they will develop the disease.

Finding out that she is antibody positive has not, so far, caused Margaret to become this anxious, though, inevitably, she worries about whether she will develop AIDS and is constantly on the alert for any signs of illness.

'I sit and look at myself. I've always suffered from mouth ulcers anyway and of course when there's an ulcer now I'm even more worried about it. I'll sit and look for ulcers and things like that. I'm also very worried about my weight. I don't like it if I lose a bit of weight. If I get anything I go to the doctor straight away. I wouldn't have done that before.'

Unfortunately, many of the symptoms of anxiety and worry – sweating, feeling feverish, diarrhoea, weight loss, fatigue – are similar to those of AIDS. A woman who is worried about her condition may therefore mistake the symptoms of stress, or a mild infection, for signs that she is developing AIDS. This may make her feel even more anxious, causing a worsening of her symptoms, which further confirms her belief that she may have the disease. It is important, for this reason, that the symptoms of anxiety are explained to women who are antibody positive soon after they are told of the test result.

Reading about AIDS in the newspaper or seeing something about it on the television can also be a source of distress and worry. One solution is to avoid the frequently inaccurate and gloomy coverage of AIDS in the media. Margaret no longer watches the news or reads a Sunday newspaper. 'I get upset if I read things in the newspaper or see something about AIDS on the television. I have a good cry. I don't believe everything I read, but it still upsets me.'

Depression

Two years after being diagnosed as antibody positive Margaret remains in good health. She keeps fit and shows no signs of developing AIDS or HIV-related illness. Despite this, and the fact that she says she has come to terms with her condition, she frequently gets depressed.

'I get depressed an awful lot. I've been depressed before, but not like this. I'll always find something on the subject to depress me. Like if I read a tiny clip in the paper I'll make a big scene over it. It's mostly at night, when I'm lying in bed. I haven't slept for about five or six nights now but I don't know why. I'm also getting really bad headaches but I don't know if it's tension or depression or what. I think it's because I'm tired and I get upset.'

This is a common reaction. Most people when they find out that they have AIDS or are antibody positive become depressed. Since AIDS is a disease which is, ultimately, fatal this is understandable. Many people with AIDS feel that they no longer have any control over their lives. Their sense of helplessness is exacerbated by the fact that not only is AIDS incurable, it also tends to run an unpredictable course. Some people die quickly whereas others may be in and out of treatment for several years, with periods of relatively good health interspersed between bouts of illness. The process of medical observation and treatment immediately following diagnosis, which inevitably disrupts a person's normal routines, can also contribute to a feeling of loss of personal control and identity. Similarly, those who have ARC or are infected with HIV may feel powerless to do anything to prevent themselves from going on to develop AIDS.

Feeling trapped and unable to do anything to change the situation, some women may become extremely despondent and lose interest in life. Activities which they previously found interesting and enjoyable start to become a chore, and they may stop going out or doing things they used to enjoy. There may be other reasons, besides feeling helpless, why someone with AIDS becomes depressed. AIDS is a physically debilitating and disfiguring disease. Many people with AIDS, especially in the latter stages of the disease, are weak and become increasingly dependent on others to look after them. They may also be in a great deal of pain and discomfort. Because of these physical limitations, a woman with AIDS may become isolated socially. Whether it is for this reason, or because of fears of how others will react, social isolation is another source of depression.

Women with AIDS or HIV who are depressed need to be encouraged to mix socially. As Margaret says, 'Lately I've been trying to get out more often to try and take my mind off things, because I think there's nothing worse than just sitting thinking.'

The preoccupation with illness and death which some women experience also makes it important to plan activities which are enjoyable. Establishing routines may also afford some distraction from anxious or depressing thoughts.

Apart from consistently feeling very low – that 'nothing's any fun any more' – someone who is depressed is likely to experience a number of other changes. They may find it difficult to concentrate, feel unable to cope even with simple tasks, lack motivation to do things, have problems sleeping, lose their appetite, and have no interest in sex.

They may also feel extremely guilty and blame themselves for all sorts of things, including their condition. Such reactions are most likely to occur when someone has caught the virus through activities which are not socially approved of. In women this usually means through injecting drugs or certain forms of sexual activity, in particular, where a woman is having sex with a number of different partners, whether for payment or not. The media portrayal of prostitutes and drug users (as well as gay men) as somehow being to blame for the spread of AIDS encourages feelings of self-recrimination and blame. While not all women will accept such definitions, those who do may experience a marked drop in self-esteem. They may also feel angry with themselves for 'causing' their condition.

The reactions of others to a diagnosis of AIDS or HIV infection can also have an important effect on a woman's self-esteem. A woman may feel like a 'social leper' as a result of being rejected by friends, lovers, family members or work colleagues. Changes in her physical appearance due to AIDS or HIV-related illness can also contribute to a loss of self-esteem.

Given the nature of the disease, and the social and financial difficulties that women with AIDS and HIV infection often have to face, suicidal feelings may also occur. It may seem that the future is so bleak that life is simply not worth living any more. Some researchers believe that relaxation and meditation techniques may help to overcome the sense of hopelessness which often signals rapid physical decline in many diagnosed as having a terminal illness. The 'Simonton method', where a person visualises from a deep state of relaxation that their white blood cells are destroying the virus, is one such technique. Teaching relaxation and imagery techniques can also be useful in the management of anxiety.

Another approach to dealing with AIDS which has clearly helped many people is to develop a healthier lifestyle, for instance by making improvements in diet, exercising regularly, lessening stress and cutting out or cutting down on alcohol, cigarettes and other drugs that are known to damage health.

Women who are antibody positive may also find such an approach useful. Margaret takes regular exercise. She goes to keep-fit, swims regularly and enjoys going for long walks. Doing all these things, she believes, helps to protect her immune system and reduces her chances of becoming ill. She also takes care of herself in other ways:

'I don't drink a lot now because I know that lowers your immune system. I eat well. Of course I'm very conscious about my weight now in case I lose weight. I don't smoke. I keep myself wrapped up in winter. For instance, when I come out of the baths I make sure that I'm extra dry and my hair is dry because I'm terrified of getting a cold.'

Whilst there is no evidence that any of these regimes can prevent or otherwise alter the course of AIDS, some researchers suspect that they may play a part in restricting the development of the disease. Certainly, they can do no harm and will increase the feeling of being in control of one's life and responsible, to a large extent, for one's own health.

Without a medical cure for AIDS many feel that

conventional medical treatment has little to offer. In this context, the therapies that are likely to improve the quality of life for people with AIDS and, most importantly, give them hope are those which encourage their efforts to help themselves.

Sexuality

Sex may be a particularly emotive subject for women who are antibody positive or have AIDS, especially if they contracted the virus this way. Equally, the restrictions on sexual contact that are recommended may be upsetting for some. Certainly this applies to Margaret. Even though she feels that in many ways knowing they are antibody positive has brought her and her husband closer together, Margaret finds these recommendations have affected their lovemaking. She and her husband also have sex less often.

'When you are in the middle of it, it's still in your mind. You can't enjoy it as much for that reason. I still very much want to make love with my husband but the virus is always on my mind. I have a good cry before sometimes, or afterwards. I can still enjoy myself, very much, but it's restrictive, especially oral sex. I don't really kiss my husband on the lips all that often any more. That's difficult because I love smoochy kisses and he won't give me one. It's just a peck usually. He's being more cautious than me.

'I think it's been more difficult for him, definitely, because if he'd known earlier, he'd have had it chopped off. That's what he's always said. If he'd have known he'd never have made love to me in the first place. That's what he's upset about, the fact that he's passed it on to me and that he didn't know. He feels so guilty.'

The knowledge that she could transmit the virus sexually is something Margaret is equally aware of. She feels that if she ever did meet someone she wanted to have sex with, besides her husband, her conscience wouldn't let her. 'I wouldn't have sex with anyone else in case I passed it on to them, even with a sheath. I don't even think I'd want to.'

For Margaret there are other worries about transmission specific to women. Anxiety about becoming pregnant is something which, to varying degrees, many women experience when they have sexual intercourse. This is especially true for Margaret. Like other women who are antibody positive she has been advised not to have children on the grounds that she might pass the virus on to the child and, also, possibly increase her own chances of developing AIDS.

While some women may not, Margaret has found this very difficult to come to terms with. This is understandable. Women are expected to want children. Indeed, there are strong social pressures on women to see motherhood as a central aspect of their lives and their self-identity. Nevertheless Margaret has, reluctantly, accepted the advice she has been given and, as she says, is anxious to avoid pregnancy. 'I worry in case anything happens. If I ever became pregnant what would I do? That's the biggest fear. I'm on the pill, as well as using the sheath.'

6 Caring for people with AIDS

While women do get AIDS, it is as carers of people with AIDS that the disease has, so far, had its biggest impact on women's lives. This is because in our society those who do most of the caring for the sick, both within the home and outside it, are women.

Caring is an activity which is seen as natural for women. This is why occupations such as nursing, looking after the elderly and work with young children are generally thought of as 'women's work'. The assumption is that women have a natural aptitude for such work that most men lack. In some situations it is also regarded as a woman's duty to care. As wives and mothers women are expected to care for their children, their husbands and both his and their own parents should they ever become ill or infirm. Such beliefs can produce feelings of guilt in women who, for whatever reasons, do not provide the care. In other cases, women may feel they have no choice but to carry on caring. This will be more likely when there is a lack of real alternatives to 'care in the community', as women's unpaid care in the home is often called.

This chapter looks at what it means to care for someone with AIDS, the dilemmas which caring poses for women, and the practical issues that can arise.

The experience of care

Finding out that someone you know has AIDS is likely to come as a tremendous shock. In many cases this is made worse by the fact that the person with AIDS has not previously said that they are gay or bisexual, or that they inject drugs.

Richard is in his early thirties, gay, and has AIDS. Though he decided not to tell his father he was gay his mother, Maggie, has known for a long time. She also knew when her son was diagnosed as antibody positive and worried when he started to lose weight and became progressively more and more exhausted. In the summer of 1986, her worst fears were confirmed. Richard developed pneumocystis and was taken into hospital. It was there that he told his mother that he had AIDS.

> 'Although you think you've prepared yourself, nothing prepares you for it. It was a *terrible* shock. Of course it was even more terrible for my husband because he'd never been actually appraised of the fact that Richard was even gay.'

Apart from the initial experience of shock most people, on learning that a friend or relative has AIDS, will suffer from the same feelings of helplessness as the person who has got AIDS. They will also feel considerable sorrow at the thought, not just of them dying, but also of the pain and suffering which they may have to endure.

Depending on how the disease was contracted, some women may also be very angry. Many men, for instance, don't tell their wives or girlfriends when they have sex with someone else, especially if it is another man. However they react, this will have an important bearing on their ability and willingness to care.

A labour of love

Caring is not just an activity, a form of work, it is also a set of feelings. When we talk about caring for someone we usually mean that we feel loving towards them and are concerned about their welfare. Caring, in this sense, is something many women want to, and expect to, provide, especially within the family.

Maggie feels this way about her son. She wants to care for him and, although she knows this will get more difficult as his condition worsens, would find it dreadful not to be able to.

> 'I think that would be the worst thing that could happen, if I couldn't physically do it, that would be terrible for me. I don't look forward to it. It fills me with fear because you don't know how you're going to cope and you don't know what you'll have to cope with either. But not being able to do anything about it would be devastating.'

However much they may want to care, many women experience an understandable tension between their own needs and those of the person being cared for. Whilst they may accept this as part of the caring role, this may involve a number of important costs to them.

> 'When I first knew Richard had AIDS I thought that's it, there's only one thing that's important and that's to be able to do whatever I can for him. So I just cleared my calendar – because I'm a terrible dabbler in this and that and I've got all sorts of strings to my bow – so that I had no commitments other than to him and to my husband. Now I keep a foothold in my outside activities, without taking on a responsibility that would be difficult to drop if I were needed.'

When her son first came out of hospital Maggie looked after him for a month. He was not bedridden, but he was very weak and frail as a result of the pneumocystis and the side-effects of the drugs used in treating it. The extra work involved in caring for him then, and since, Maggie has not found difficult. 'After all, between looking after two and looking after three is not a lot of difference really.' In her case the stresses and strains of caring are associated with the emotional aspects of providing care.

'When you're actually coping with the worst parts of it, it's as if you've got some sort of power inside of you that keeps you going, keeps you putting on your make-up and making sure that you're looking good when you see them and, when you go to the hospital, that you're not down-hearted. But then, afterwards, you get very tired, terribly tired and for no good reason it seems. You just feel dreadfully tired.'

Those providing support and friendship to people with AIDS are in an unpredictable situation. Some people who have AIDS die suddenly, others may be in and out of treatment for several years. The uncertainty of knowing how the illness will progress can cause a great deal of stress, both for people with AIDS and for their carers. In addition, those providing care share the difficulty of knowing how best to respond to someone whose mood is likely to fluctuate between hope and despair.

'The stresses I find are not knowing what's going on inside him and knowing how far to push and how far not to push. For instance I would like to be much more demonstrative, but I hesitate. I suppose I'm looking for reassurance from him. I have no fear of him, but because I am so anxious about him I want to smother him and you can't do that. You see everything you do is two-edged in a way. You don't want to remind him that he's ill, and you don't want him to think that you're being crass. So you're walking a tightrope really.'

Although Maggie does not, many women caring for someone within the home feel isolated and cut off from the outside world. This is likely to be particularly true of women who receive little or no support as carers. The decision whether or not to tell others will therefore be important in terms of how women caring for people with AIDS experience their caring role.

In Maggie's case, she felt that she had to tell many of her friends. This was partly because she didn't want them to think she was putting them at risk, especially those who had young children. 'A lot of them knew Richard was gay and, although they hadn't said it, when he got ill I know a lot of them suspected he had AIDS.'

Her decision was also based on how she thought she would be able to cope with the situation.

'I felt totally selfish about it. I thought this is my situation and I've got to cope with it the best way I can, and if I lose friends well I've just got to lose them. In fact, I've had a lot of support from my friends, they have been wonderful about it. Mind you I haven't told everybody, I've been selective. Some people are just bigotted and you don't tell them.'

Although she feels extremely fortunate in her friends, and has been relieved and comforted by the sympathy and support which they have offered her, a few have reacted with fear and prejudice.

'Some who don't like the idea of anybody being gay have been less than sympathetic, and one or two have actually kept away. They don't want to come to the house because there's infection here. I'm sorry to lose people in that way but that's their decision. I am, I suppose, resentful about it in a way, and disappointed, but it's something you've got to put up with.'

The fear of developing AIDS is something that carers of people with AIDS may also experience. A woman whose husband or lover has AIDS, for instance, is particularly likely to feel anxious. Not only will she probably be worried about what will happen to her partner, but she will also be thinking, 'Will I get it?' In some cases the stresses this can put on a relationship may be too much, and it may end. Alternatively, the experience of dealing with these sorts of anxieties may, in other situations, bring two people closer together.

The possibility of contracting the virus is something that has never really worried Maggie. She knows enough about AIDS to understand that, with a few simple precautions, caring for her son does not put her at risk. Her anxieties are for her son and his health.

> 'You don't really take it all in at first. It isn't until you begin to think about it that the whole implications come to you and you just get *more* anxious. Every nuance of health of your son you're tending to be. . . . It's a dreadful thing to say, but you're almost waiting for the worst.'

Maggie does not always feel like this. As she says, 'You swing from hope to despair. Both feelings are true, but it's very important to encourage people to be hopeful.'

Apart from the uncertainty of how his illness will progress, there is also the worry for Maggie that she may put her son at risk by passing on germs and diseases.

> 'I had a bad cold so I decided although I was going to see him I wouldn't, because I was at the infectious stage and it's silly to court trouble. He's living an ordinary life and obviously he's going to come up against ordinary germs, but I wouldn't push him into any infectious situation.'

It is important that lovers, as well as friends and

How can I help if someone I know has AIDS?

First of all you can find out about AIDS. Some people with AIDS, or who are antibody positive, have lost friends because they are misinformed or do not understand about how the virus is transmitted. Because they may be afraid of losing friends, a person who has HIV or AIDS needs to know who they can rely on. It is important to reassure them that you are not afraid and that you know you can't get AIDS by simply befriending someone who has it. There are many ways of doing this. For instance Maggie's daughter 'took the children when she visited Richard because she wanted to reassure him that she had no fears of him.' It is also important to show affection and to touch. Like anyone else, someone who is antibody positive or has AIDS needs physical contact and will, also, enjoy the reassurance that goes with it.

The fear many people have of AIDS is likely to have a big impact on a person's self-esteem and confidence. They may be reluctant to tell others they have AIDS, or the virus which causes it, or to discuss their diagnosis. Show them that if they want to talk about their illness you are willing to listen. Try to understand if they become angry and frustrated, and don't be afraid to talk about how you feel. What is important is that someone who has AIDS has friends with whom they feel they can be honest and at ease.

When someone is not well they may not always feel up to talking. Try to be aware of this and the limits that being ill, as well as often feeling miserable and depressed, can put on a person's social life. Let them know when you intend to visit and don't be offended if they don't want you to stay for very long. People who are ill often tire easily.

People with AIDS progress through their illness at vastly different rates and with varying degrees of ability to continue their daily activities. Offer practical help if you are able, and if you can't visit try to phone or write. A person who is well may require sudden hospitalisation and even die. *Keep in touch.*

relatives of people with AIDS, have the opportunity to discuss their anxieties about what a diagnosis of AIDS means and the risk of infection to themselves. They need to know what precautions they should take. They also need to be aware of what is likely to happen, both physically and psychologically, to someone who has AIDS as the disease progresses, and of what they can do to help. When a person with AIDS dies, bereavement counselling is also often needed.

Counselling for families, friends and lovers is available at some hospitals and STD clinics (see page 138). A woman who is, or may end up, caring for someone with AIDS may also find it useful to join a self-help group.

Though she says she probably wouldn't go along until her son's condition became much worse, Maggie feels it would help her to talk to women in a similar situation.

'Although one thinks one is staunchly independent there are all sorts of things I realise I need. I do need support. Also, you want to know what's going on for other people and, you know, one's weaknesses are not so crushing if you find someone else is just as weak.'

There are a number of groups already in existence for parents of people with AIDS. For information about these and other organisations giving information and advice about AIDS see pages 137-41.

Caring means work

Caring for someone who has AIDS can be hard work. Although people with AIDS may experience periods of relatively good health during which they are able to continue their daily activities, there will also be times when they cannot manage by themselves. Basic everyday tasks such as cooking a meal, shopping, cleaning and doing the laundry have to be done for them. They may be bedridden, especially in the latter stages of the disease, too ill or too weak to wash, feed themselves or even go to the toilet alone.

Usually it is women – as daughters, wives and mothers – who are expected to provide this care. The medical profession, social services staff and the person who is ill may all assume this. They may also take it for granted that however difficult the circumstances a woman will cope. Very rarely are women asked if they feel able to take on board the care of a sick or elderly relative. Nor are they usually asked what help and support they will need to enable them to do the job of caring.

Because of these expectations women, unlike men, can be under considerable pressure to give up a job to care for someone. Women who do give up paid work to become a 'full-time' carer may find it extremely difficult to adjust to being financially dependent on someone else or on state benefits. They may also experience considerable isolation, especially if very few people know about the diagnosis. Equally, the strain on women who, by choice or necessity, combine going out to work with providing this kind of physical care can be enormous. Apart from the demands on her time and energy, a woman may feel very anxious or guilty about continuing working.

The provision of services such as home helps, day care centres, meals on wheels, and short-term places in residential homes could reduce the stresses experienced by women caring for people with AIDS, whether working outside the home or not. Although women's access to such services will vary, many women will not get the practical support they need.

For women who, like Maggie, do want to provide care in the home but who also recognise that they may need some help, this is an important issue.

'I would like to see an availability, a possibility of getting help in the home, most decidedly I would. I think it's terrible if they can't be coped with at home.

Basically it should just be a part of health care. It should
be as easy to get help when it's necessary whether it's
AIDS or anything else, but it's not likely to be because
of the fear of it, in the home anyway, and of course in
some hospitals too. It will have to have vast resources
allocated to it.'

In the present climate this seems unlikely. Whilst
emphasising the importance of 'care in the community',
the government is committed to spending less and less on
health and social services. Apart from the effects this will
have on women caring for people with AIDS as 'a labour
of love', this will place an increasing strain on those
whose job it is to care.

Women doing AIDS work

Health workers will have to confront their own feelings of
sorrow and hopelessness which can result from working
with the fatally ill. While most of us develop a certain
acceptance of death in the elderly and infirm, few people
find it easy to deal with a young person who is dying.
The fact that AIDS is a disfiguring and debilitating disease
makes it even harder to accept.

The risk of infection is something else which those who
provide care for people with AIDS, or the much larger
number who are antibody positive, are likely to be
concerned about. This is an understandable concern given
the nature of the disease. Nevertheless, it would seem
that the risks are small. There has not been a single case
of a health care worker developing AIDS as a result of
their work.

The most likely way in which HIV may be transmitted
to medical and nursing staff is through needle-stick
injury. This has already happened in England. A nurse
who sustained a serious needle-stick injury, which
involved the injection of a small amount of blood from an

AIDS patient, later developed antibodies to the virus. However, the risk of infection from such accidents seems to be low. Studies both in the United Kingdom and in the United States indicate that in almost all cases where hospital staff have been accidentally exposed to blood or bodily fluids of people infected with HIV, the antibody test is negative.

Although the evidence is that HIV is not easily transmitted to those who care for people with AIDS, certain precautions do need to be taken.

The main precautions are those which are necessary to avoid coming into contact with bodily fluids. There is no need, for instance, for hospital staff to wear gloves and masks just to enter an AIDS patient's room, as has sometimes happened. Apart from being unnecessary, this is likely to upset both the person with AIDS and their visitors.

Guidelines for health care workers have been drawn up outlining ways of reducing the risk of infection (see, for example, the report of the Advisory Committee on Dangerous Pathogens, 1986 and the Report of the Royal College of Nursing AIDS Working Party, 1986). Among the measures recommended is the careful handling of needles and sharp instruments. The majority of self-inoculation accidents can be avoided by not resheathing needles. Needles should either be thrown away on the syringe or, if this is not possible, removed from syringes without resheathing them and disposed of in a suitable container. Where there is a risk of coming into contact with blood or other bodily fluids which may contain the virus, disposable rubber gloves and a plastic apron should be worn. The membranes of the eyes and mouth may allow transmission of the virus, and where there is a risk of splashing of fluid which may contain HIV eye and mouth protection is advisable.

In addition to knowing about the nature of the disease, how HIV is transmitted and how the risk of this happening can be reduced, health care workers also need to be aware of the psychological implications of being diagnosed as having AIDS. This is especially true of nurses. Because they are more closely involved with patients, they have a potentially important role to play in providing emotional support as well as physical care.

This can be stressful. Most likely, someone who has AIDS will feel depressed and anxious. They may need to talk about their illness, including their fears about death and dying. They may also feel very angry about the effects of having AIDS, and may take out their anger and frustration on hospital staff. This may be true of relatives and friends who, in addition, may ask difficult and often upsetting questions. A nurse may also have to confront issues that she has never had to deal with before such as, for instance, her own and other people's reactions to gay relationships.

Training programmes for people providing AIDS-related services, both paid and voluntary, should include information and advice on how to deal with these kind of situations. Also, in addition to developing an understanding of the needs of people with AIDS and those affected by the diagnosis, it may be useful for workers to examine their own attitudes towards death and dying. In view of the fact that in this country the majority of those who have AIDS are gay men, it is also important to have some knowledge of gay lifestyles. Negative attitudes and judgments regarding gay lifestyles are not uncommon, and will need to be challenged. Health workers should also realise that many AIDS patients experience painful consequences when entering a health care system designed for and administered by a predominantly heterosexual population. Visiting regulations, for instance, may not recognise gay relationships as being as important as other relationships. Wherever possible hospital staff should take steps to prevent this and other forms of discrimination from occurring.

Discrimination can have other implications for care providers. Most gay or bisexual men are careful who they tell about their sexuality. It is vitally important therefore that staff remember who does and does not know. Even when someone is not gay, the stigma surrounding AIDS makes considentiality a major issue. Those working with people who have AIDS or are antibody positive should not disclose information about diagnosis unless the person wants or has agreed to this. The issue of confidentiality is discussed in more detail on page 127.

The stresses on women caring for people with AIDS are made worse by consistent underspending within the NHS and on social services. Without the money to employ more staff, those whose job it is to provide physical and psychological care will increasingly be under pressure as the number of people who have AIDS grows.

It may be helpful to have a support group for those working with people with AIDS where there is the opportunity to discuss some of the stresses, as well as the practical problems, that can arise. What is really needed, however, is a change in governmental policy to meet the growing costs of AIDS.

Carers of children with AIDS

As of November 1986, 376 cases of AIDS in children had been reported in the United States. In Africa, where women get AIDS almost as often as men, the figures are much higher. In contrast to this, only six children in the UK have AIDS, and relatively few so far have the virus (August 1986).

This is likely to change as more infants are born to women who are antibody positive or have AIDS. As I described in Chapter 2, women infected with HIV may transmit the virus to their infants during pregnancy or birth or possibly through breast milk. It is not yet known what proportion of children who contract the virus from their mothers are likely to go on to develop AIDS, though some doctors have suggested that it may be as many as half.

Women who have AIDS or HIV infection are currently being advised against having children or, if they are already pregnant, to have an abortion. This is not only because of the possible risk to the baby. In women with HIV infection, pregnancy may also possibly increase their own chances of going on to develop AIDS.

The other main way in which children get AIDS is through having a blood or blood product transfusion. This includes children with haemophilia, almost all of whom are male, who receive treatment with the blood clotting agents factor 8 and factor 9. Of the 700 or so children who have haemophilia in the UK most have now been tested for HIV. About a third of these are antibody positive. They contracted the virus as a result of the blood products used in treatment being infected with HIV. Fortunately the risk of this happening in future has been largely eliminated through the screening of blood donors and heat treatment of factor 8 and factor 9. The number of children with haemophilia who are infected with HIV will therefore gradually diminish as these children reach school-leaving age.

The types of opportunistic infections in infants are different from those seen in adults with AIDS. Although there are some cases of opportunistic infections such as pneumocystis and oral thrush, other infections such as meningitis are more common. Kaposi's sarcoma is rare.

Even though they may be expecting it, being told that their child has AIDS, or the virus which can lead to AIDS, will be enormously distressing for most women. There are, for instance, the emotional problems associated with knowing that they may be caring for a child with a limited lifespan. They may also be extremely anxious about not only their own risk of developing AIDS, but also about their child's health.

If their child does become ill and develop AIDS they may feel very guilty that it is their fault. This may apply to mothers of children with haemophilia as well as, more obviously, to women who have transmitted the virus to their infants. Knowing that she is a carrier of haemo-philia, a woman may blame herself for passing on the disease which has put her child at risk.

Some women will be anxious about other people finding out that their child is antibody positive or has AIDS. One of the reasons for not wanting anyone to know is in case one's child becomes stigmatised. For example, some parents, fearing that their own child might be at risk of infection, have demanded that children with HIV should be removed from schools. At another level, other children might refuse to mix or play with a child who is known to be infected with the virus.

There is, in fact, no evidence to show that children with HIV transmit the virus to other members of their family, friends or teachers through normal social contact such as occurs in schools. Children who have the virus can safely attend school without putting other children at risk. It is important that parents understand this. In addition, schools should make sure that both staff and pupils know how HIV is transmitted.

To prevent AIDS discrimination it is advisable to tell as few people as possible that one's child is infected with HIV or has AIDS. Those who do know, especially teachers, should be aware of the need for confidentiality *and should tell no one*, unless they have permission from the child's parents to do so. Most haemophilia centres do not tell schools which of the children they treat are sero-positive (antibody positive). They take the view that teachers should know, in any case, how to deal with a bleeding injury if a child in their care is known to have haemophilia and, possibly, HIV. The decision not to tell others may be difficult to explain to a child. As one woman said, it's hard to explain to them that although having HIV or AIDS is nothing to be ashamed of, this is something to be kept a secret.

Children who are antibody positive or have AIDS need to have as normal a life as possible. At school they should be treated in the same way as other pupils. Nevertheless,

there are a few precautions which a woman caring for a
child with HIV infection or AIDS needs to take in order to
protect both herself and her child. Some of these are
listed below. Further information on reducing the risk
of infection, especially within schools, is contained in
the DES booklet *Children at School: Problems Related to
AIDS*.

It is not only those who care for children with AIDS,
within the home and at school, who need to be informed.
In America children with AIDS or HIV have created
enormous public policy problems concerning not only
schools, but also adoption and fostering for children
whose mothers are too ill to care for them or who die

Caring for children who are antibody positive or have AIDS

- Any spills should be cleaned up using household bleach
  diluted one in ten with water.
- Urine, faeces and vomit may contain blood. Wear
  disposable rubber gloves when cleaning these up, and
  cover any cuts on your hands with waterproof plasters.
- Dirty nappies should be burnt, flushed down the toilet
  or put in a sealed plastic bag. Non-disposable nappies
  and clothes or linen that are stained with blood, urine,
  vomit or faeces should be washed in the hottest cycle of
  a washing machine or boiled.
- Women who are antibody positive or have AIDS should
  not breastfeed their children.
- Because the virus is transmitted in blood it is important
  to discourage practices such as tattooing and ear-
  piercing, which some children may engage in. Cover any
  cuts or grazes on either yourself or your child with
  waterproof plasters.
- Children with AIDS or HIV infection have the same need
  for affection as other children. There is no risk in
  hugging or cuddling them.

because of AIDS or are unable to care for their children for other reasons. In this country, health and social service providers are beginning to have to deal with these issues. The following chapter examines this and other aspects of AIDS policy making in more detail, and asks the question, 'What can be done?'

7 Policies and prevention

While health care providers and volunteers cope with the realities of dealing with those who have the disease, policy makers have, until recently, done little to halt the spread of AIDS. Undoubtedly, if AIDS had initially affected a different social group to gay men then the situation would have been different. As long as the disease was confined largely to gay men the British government did very little. In 1985, for instance, less than £5 million was spent on AIDS. It is only the recognition that AIDS poses a serious threat to the heterosexual as well as to the gay community that has prompted the government to take AIDS more seriously and, alongside this, provide more funding. In 1986 the government announced it was to spend a further £10 million on public education alone.

Funding nevertheless remains an urgent priority, especially for the treatment and care of those who have already been infected with HIV. In addition to providing more money for AIDS programmes, the government must also examine the wider social implications of AIDS, in particular, the need for legislation to prevent discrimination against people with AIDS, or who are antibody positive, in employment, health care delivery, housing and education.

Education

The three major areas which need funding are prevention campaigns, health and social service programmes for people with AIDS, and research aimed at developing a cure and vaccine. In America, governmental efforts have focused on finding a vaccine to protect people who do not have AIDS from getting it. The government has neglected to provide adequate funding either for the medical treatment and care of those who are ill or dying from AIDS or for education.

The British experience is a few years behind that of the United States. Britain has, therefore, the opportunity to learn from its mistakes, and to take the necessary steps to try to prevent the AIDS epidemic from reaching the same proportions.

Clearly, it was a mistake that education was the least well planned component of AIDS prevention measures in the United States. A vaccine has not yet been developed and probably won't be until the 1990s at the earliest. Even if a vaccine is produced, it may not offer the ultimate solution. One of the characteristics of HIV is that it is constantly changing and producing new strains. A vaccine which is effective against one strain may not be against another. (Some of the problems in developing a vaccine are discussed on page 23.)

In the absence of a vaccine or a cure, public education is the most effective way of preventing the spread of AIDS. Apart from the human suffering which AIDS causes, attempts to halt the disease also make good economic sense when one considers the cost of providing AIDS-related services. Thousands of pounds spent on education now could save millions of pounds on medical treatment and care in the future.

However, what we must remember is that AIDS unites things which society is reluctant to talk about: homo-sexuality, sexual disease and death. In addition to this, the much-needed explicit advice about safe sex may be resisted because it involves discussing activities that some people consider 'deviant' or offensive.

In the United States concern about how the public would react to widespread discussion of, in particular, gay sex and drug use has fundamentally influenced attitudes towards education campaigns. In Los Angeles the State Department of Health Services issued a directive to halt distribution of an AIDS prevention brochure aimed at gay men almost as soon as the governor's office learned of it. The pamphlet, *Mother's Handy Sex Guide*, advised gay men about safer sex practices and was part of the high-profile 'LA Cares' mass media campaign launched in 1985. Another brochure aimed at encouraging gay men to adopt safer sexual practices was attacked by one LA county supervisor as 'hard core pornographic trash, totally unsuitable for the public'.

If we in Britain are to learn anything from such reactions, it is that they should be avoided at all costs. The *only* way for individuals to protect themselves from getting AIDS is to know how HIV may be transmitted and to take steps to reduce the risk of this happening. For some this will mean a significant change in social and sexual attitudes. AIDS education, if it is to be effective, must tackle this. It must, for example, challenge the widely held belief, especially amongst men, that every road to ultimate sexual satisfaction must end in intercourse, as this is a way of transmitting the virus.

So far the government has been slow to respond to the need for educational programmes aimed at preventing the spread of AIDS. Until 1986, the provision of information for those at risk, and the general public, was left largely to voluntary organisations such as the Terrence Higgins Trust and the Haemophilia Society.

In March 1986 the government launched a £2½ million public information campaign on how to avoid AIDS. This included material specifically designed for people at risk as well as information directed at the general public.

Advertisements entitled 'Don't Aid AIDS' were placed in both the national newspapers and, after some deliberation, the gay press. Bearing a government warning that the facts 'may shock, but should not offend', the ads sought to inform and reassure people about the spread of AIDS and offered some broad guidelines about safe sex. A leaflet giving more detailed advice, and a telephone information service providing recorded information, were also part of the campaign.

As a start, this was a welcome sign that at last the government was beginning to take AIDS prevention seriously. However, a real commitment to halting the spread of AIDS requires that much more money be spent on health education. The message to be learned from the American experience is quite simple. The longer we wait the more AIDS cases we are likely to have. One of the problems with the long incubation period for AIDS is that governments may not respond until there is a large number of cases of AIDS. By then the number of people infected with the virus is already quite high. The government must act now, by providing adequate funding for AIDS prevention in the form of public education that is both comprehensive and explicit.

A good example of public education on AIDS is found in San Francisco. The city's programme includes advertisements on public transport and TV and in newspapers and magazines, and news and feature stories, as well as explicit leaflets for groups at risk. While the efforts of voluntary organisations such as the San Francisco AIDS Foundation and the Shanti Project have been enormously important, such developments also reflect the willingness of the city government to become involved in attempts to prevent the spread of AIDS. San Francisco has provided more direct support to AIDS programmes than any other city in the United States.

Apart from a dramatic increase in government spending, what is also needed in the UK is a change in educational policy towards the teaching of sexual, including homosexual, material if AIDS prevention is to succeed. At the moment there is little if any discussion of homosexuality in many schools and colleges, where sex education is frequently based around discussions of heterosexual intercourse.

Young people must be given information about AIDS and how it is spread so that they become aware of the risks associated with certain kinds of sex and also of experimenting with injecting drugs. Education in schools is therefore vital, and must include explicit discussion of sexuality in the broadest sense. Unfortunately, this would seem unlikely to be an outcome of the recent Education Bill. The Bill gives parents the right to decide whether their child receives sex education in school and governors the right to decide what that education should be.

AIDS education is essential not only as a form of disease prevention, but also as a means of combating the fear and ignorance surrounding the disease. This, in combination with anti-gay attitudes, helps explain why some people with AIDS have experienced a hostile or unsympathetic response from others. The mass media, which have a potentially important role to play in AIDS education, must take some responsibility for this. Indeed, the approach of certain sections of the media has been both sensationalising and judgmental. This kind of media coverage has done absolutely nothing to allay people's irrational fears, in particular that AIDS is a casually spread disease. It is not.

It is vital that this is widely understood, especially by those who have to care for people with AIDS. Yet even amongst health care workers it would appear that fears about catching HIV through routine contact with AIDS patients do exist. Such fears can result in decreased quality of care to people with AIDS. There have, for instance, been cases of hospital staff refusing to feed or wash a patient if they have AIDS. Similarly, some doctors have told their patients not to come back to their surgery if they have AIDS.

Such examples only serve to underline the importance of providing education programmes for health authority staff, of all grades. More generally, it is essential that we all learn to recognise the *real* risks of getting AIDS and how to protect against them.

Health and social services

Health education is not the only AIDS-related policy issue that we urgently need to consider. The provision of funds for health and social services programmes for those with AIDS and HIV-related conditions is also a major area of concern, particularly as the number of cases of AIDS reported seems to be doubling approximately every 10 months. (By the end of 1985 273 cases had been reported in the United Kingdom. By October 1986 this figure had increased to 548.)

Despite this, the service needs of people with AIDS have not been considered funding priorities. On the contrary, the health and social services found themselves having to cope with AIDS at a time when the government was committed to making major cuts in spending. Apart from the strain which this has placed on the medical and welfare services that already exist, this has had direct effects on the care and treatment of people with AIDS.

The situation will worsen as more people develop AIDS, unless the government provides funding for the expansion in services that is urgently needed. This has particular implications for women. The health system is already biased against the needs of women, especially those who are poor, black or who may possibly be at risk of AIDS through injecting drugs or prostitution.

Improved care and access to support, both in and out of hospital, is perhaps the most pressing need for AIDS patients. In the case of hospital and medical care of people with AIDS this means more hospital beds, more equipment and more staff to meet the increased workload generated by AIDS patients.

An alternative to hospital care is the kind of care offered by the hospice movement to the terminally ill. Hospice care could play an increasingly important role in the care and treatment of people with AIDS. Again, this will depend on whether funding is available. Further government spending on the training of health workers in caring for patients with AIDS is also needed. Research on the development of therapies to treat those who have already been infected with HIV also remains in urgent need of government support.

Apart from hospital care, which is enormously costly, more support services are needed to enable people with AIDS to be cared for at home if that is what they want. A person with AIDS may be too ill to cook a meal for themselves or do the housework or shopping. They may not even be able to get out of bed on their own. Home-help programmes and improved hospital out-patients services are therefore necessary, if people with AIDS are to be cared for within the community. More health and social workers trained in counselling people with AIDS will also be needed to provide emotional support and help when dealing with the many difficult issues that a diagnosis of AIDS, or HIV infection, raises. This will include dealing with the reactions of friends, family and lovers.

At present, the National Health Service is severely strained in caring for the sick. In the context of further cuts in NHS spending, this is likely to place a greater burden for AIDS care on the 'community'. As I have already pointed out, what this often means is women providing the care. All too often social policy makers, in arguing for community care, fail to acknowledge this. This must not happen with AIDS. Arguments for community care policies for people with AIDS must recognise the costs to carers, especially where few support services for carers are available. While there may be good grounds for caring for people with AIDS within the community, this must not be at the expense of women.

Apart from caring for the sick and the elderly, the role of caring for children is a traditional one for women. While this may be a very rewarding experience, for some women the conditions in which they have to care for children can mean stress, exhaustion, loneliness or boredom. Such feelings very often arise from the tremendous responsibility attached to being a mother. This reflects men's lack of involvement in child care. It also highlights the lack of social service provision for women with young children, in particular the provision of adequate day care facilities.

Women who have children with AIDS are likely to find caring for their children particularly stressful. This will be especially true of those women who themselves have AIDS or are antibody positive. A woman who is too ill to care for her children may be forced to have them taken into care. Alternatively, women who are still healthy but have passed the virus on to their child may have to deal with their child developing AIDS and dying.

Children with AIDS create enormous social policy problems concerning day care and schools, fostering and adoption for children whose mothers die or become ill, and combating AIDS discrimination. These are issues which governments will in future have to deal with. In the United States, where there are more cases of AIDS in children than in the UK, AIDS workers have begun to recognise this. In New York, for instance, the Gay Men's Health Crisis, a volunteer organisation, runs a programme directed at children with AIDS. The volunteers visit the children at home or in hospital, and also assist the family in receiving social services and home care attendants. Also in New York, a special foster care programme for children with AIDS has been developed. Apart from needing more nurseries, increased child benefits, better housing and welfare, women with young children are also very often in need of emotional support and help. In the case of women whose children have AIDS, this means providing counselling and other forms of social support.

Counselling and advisory services for those at risk are also needed. Some women may be anxious to know if they have been infected with HIV and will need counselling about whether or not they should take the antibody test. Further counselling will be needed if they decide to take the test and it turns out to be positive. Because of the possible risks to the woman and her child if she became pregnant, this should include comprehensive advice about contraception and abortion, as well as ways of reducing the risk of infection to others through safer sex and safer drug use.

At present, voluntary organisations like the Terrence Higgins Trust, the Haemophilia Society and drug advice agencies are helping to meet some of the deficiencies in the health and welfare systems. They provide information for at-risk groups and the general public, as well as offering support and counselling to those with AIDS, or who are antibody positive, and their partners and families. The Terrence Higgins Trust, for example, runs support groups for people with AIDS and who are antibody positive. The Trust also provides 'buddies' for people with AIDS. These are workers who volunteer to provide practical help and emotional support to someone with AIDS, or who is antibody positive, on a regular basis. Body Positive is another self-help organisation which runs support groups for people who have taken the HIV antibody test and are positive.

Most of these groups are for gay or bisexual men. This reflects the fact that so far it is mainly they who have been affected by AIDS. Where support groups for women do exist, these tend to be for women who are caring for someone with AIDS. The addresses of some of the organisations which offer help for parents are given on pages 137-8.

As more women develop AIDS it will become necessary to provide counselling and support services for them. Last year the Terrence Higgins Trust started its first support group for women. The Trust can also arrange for a woman worker to visit on a similar basis to the 'buddy' scheme.

Whilst governmental support of volunteer agencies like the Terrence Higgins Trust is important, and must continue, this needs to be in conjunction with increased spending in the public sector. The provision of health and social services will be severely challenged by AIDS. It is vital that government planners and policy makers recognise this, and provide long-term financing to meet the growing costs of caring for and treating those who have the disease.

Housing

In common with a significant proportion of the population of the United Kingdom, many people with AIDS are dependent on state benefits. In some cases this is because they are too ill to work. In others it is because they have lost their job as a result of their employer finding out they have AIDS. Whatever the reason, such financial hardship is likely to lead to problems with paying a mortgage or rent.

Housing can pose serious difficulties for other reasons. Some people with AIDS have been evicted when their landlords have discovered their illness, or have lost their home when their lover, friends or family have refused to continue to support them.

A woman with AIDS, or who is antibody positive, who becomes homeless can apply for local authority housing and be accepted as a priority for housing under the terms of the Housing (Homeless Persons) Act. However this may not be easy, and in some cases it may take a lot of effort to get the council to do anything. Even then, the kind of accommodation offered may be unsuitable. Very often the homeless are housed in poor quality accommodation, which may be damp or difficult to heat.

It is vital that local authorities become more aware of

the housing problems faced by people with AIDS. Apart from access to accommodation that is suitable to their needs, it is important that people with AIDS are housed quickly. For this to be possible housing agencies, together with voluntary organisations, need to develop housing programmes with AIDS in mind.

In San Francisco, voluntary organisations like the Shanti Project, with government money and support, are able to provide low-cost housing for people made homeless through AIDS. Only people with AIDS live in the houses, whose location is kept secret to protect the privacy of those living there. Each person has her or his own bedroom and shares the kitchen, bathroom and living room facilities with the other residents. Shanti also provides home care services for those who are ill to help them stay in their own home rather than go into hospital, if that is what they want.

The experience of San Francisco suggests a model for care which Britain could learn a great deal from. The housing problems of those with AIDS or who are antibody positive are not simply about having somewhere stable to live. They are also about being able to choose the kind of accommodation they want. At present, the range of choices available to people with AIDS is very limited. Housing programmes specifically designed to meet the needs of people with AIDS, such as Shanti's, remain in urgent need of government support. Further long-term financing is needed to meet the costs of providing more hospital beds and hospice facilities, as well as out-patient services and community care for those who prefer to remain in their own homes. There is also likely to be a growing demand for mental health hostel places and sheltered housing, associated with the tendency of HIV to cause early dementia, in some cases, due to brain damage.

AIDS discrimination – the antibody test

For what purposes should the government permit the use of blood tests to determine the presence of antibodies to HIV? Should they allow the test to be used to screen applicants for medical insurance or for immigration or employment? Should they use it to screen travellers from other countries where AIDS is epidemic? (Accusations of racial discrimination have already been levelled at the British government for suggesting compulsory screening of African visitors to Britain.) If the use of testing is to be promoted for the control of infection, how should this be done? Should people in high-risk groups be required to submit to HIV testing?

In the UK the HIV antibody test is used to screen blood that is donated. It is also used to screen semen and donors of kidneys, hearts, livers, etc. Opinions differ as to whether, in addition, it is appropriate to use the test to screen *people*. (This already occurs in the United States, where the HIV antibody test is given to all members of the armed forces.) A major concern is that this may lead to new forms of social control of women. Will HIV testing soon become part of routine antenatal care for instance? The development of a test for HIV infection also makes the introduction of compulsory screening of prostitutes a possibility. Similar fears that the antibody test might be used to single out gay men should also not be regarded as groundless.

A common argument for routine screening is that it would help control the spread of AIDS. Those who were antibody positive could be advised on how to reduce the risk of transmitting the virus to others. The assumption is that a person will be more likely to alter their behaviour if they know whether they are positive or negative than if they do not know. While some people may find it easier to change their lifestyle if they know the test result, the advice is the same whether they are positive or negative:

practise safer sex to avoid contracting the virus and, in the case of those who are sero-positive, passing it on to others. Consequently, many AIDS workers argue that there is little to be gained from taking the test.

A more extreme 'AIDS control' measure is the suggestion that people with AIDS, or those having tested positive on the HIV antibody test, could be quarantined. Given the irrational fears and prejudices which surround AIDS it is perhaps not surprising that the idea of isolating those who have AIDS or HIV should have occurred. However, as a public health measure this is neither realistic nor appropriate. HIV is comparatively difficult to catch, and only major changes in public policy could bring about a quarantine of the many thousands of people who are by now infected with the virus. It is through public education and counselling on safer sex and drug use that the spread of AIDS will hopefully be halted.

Another reason for limiting the use of tests is that it can be detrimental for a person to know that they are HIV positive. Many people are shocked by the news and become anxious or depressed. This is why it is essential that counselling is available both before and after the test.

While counselling can often help to overcome psychological difficulties, people who are antibody positive can have other problems. For instance, some people have lost their jobs once it was discovered that they were sero-positive. There are then often financial and accommodation problems. Sometimes people who are antibody positive have been denied medical treatment. Insurance companies are reluctant to give health or life insurance to anyone who is sero-positive. This can make it difficult to get a mortgage.

The AIDS hysteria generated by the media is partly to blame for this. However, discrimination against people with AIDS and those who are antibody positive is also connected with the fact that in the public imagination AIDS is linked with homosexuality. To a large extent, it is homophobia and anti-lesbianism, not AIDS, that's the root of the problem.

In the UK, there are at present no laws specifically designed to protect the rights of people with AIDS or those who are antibody positive. (In the United States, California has legislated confidentiality, anonymity and anti-discrimination safeguards. By contrast, Colorado was the first state to make reporting of names of people who test positive compulsory by law.) Under such conditions, confidentiality is a major issue. Many people are tested at STD clinics which are governed by special regulations to guarantee anonymity. These regulations require that, when a disease has been sexually transmitted, a health worker may not disclose information to anyone not involved in the treatment of the patient without their permission. Clinical records are also kept separate from the main hospital records which tend to be less confidential.

If a person has been referred by their GP the clinic may wish to inform them of the test result. This may have serious consequences if the GP is not sufficiently aware of the need for confidentiality, or feels it necessary to mention the result in medical reports for employers and insurance companies. A doctor may also feel it is her or his duty to tell someone that their sexual partner has AIDS or is antibody positive. Whilst it may not be general clinical practice, the British Medical Association has ruled that doctors should have the right to inform someone that their partner is antibody positive, or has AIDS, to prevent the spread of infection.

It is not enough for doctors to say they won't tell anyone if a patient has AIDS or is antibody positive. They should be prohibited by law from releasing names without good reason. Failure to implement measures to ensure confidentiality will mean continued difficulties for people who have AIDS or are antibody positive. Some may even put their lives at risk because they are afraid to go to their doctor in case their virus status becomes known.

At present, given the limitations of the tests available

and the discrimination which exists towards people with AIDS and who are antibody positive, the use of the HIV antibody test should be carefully controlled. It must be used to screen blood and semen that is donated, and for research, but it should not be used to screen people, particularly without their 'informed consent'. (We need to recognise of course that there are all sorts of ways in which someone may feel forced to 'consent'.) Bearing this in mind, the test should be widely and freely available for those who wish to use it. For instance, women in high-risk groups who are thinking about becoming pregnant or are in the early stages of pregnancy may benefit from having the test done (see pages 47-51). However it is essential that they be counselled about whether or not to continue the pregnancy as well as the social, economic, employment and emotional consequences of a positive test result *before* taking the test.

8 The challenge of AIDS

AIDS legitimises prejudices already embedded in our society. Right-wing moralists, for example, regard AIDS as proof that their values, based on traditional Christian beliefs, are correct. In their view sex outside marriage, and sex with someone of the same sex, is morally wrong. AIDS is a recognition of this, a punishment from God for society's 'acceptance' of homosexuality, prostitution and promiscuity.

AIDS could also bring about enormous changes in how people view sexuality. The notion of safe sex forces us to question many of the assumptions we hold about sex. It demands that we re-evaluate forms of sex that are often considered 'second-best'. It challenges the belief that people, but more especially men, have little voluntary control over their sexual desires (a belief that is frequently reflected in attitudes towards rape, prostitution and pornography). It encourages the development of new meanings for sex and the erotic which are not focused on intercourse, or on necessarily having an orgasm.

The assumption, very often, is that such changes in sexual attitudes and behaviour will be difficult for most of us. Safe sex will have to be sold to people as fun, exciting and satisfying before they will want to practise it.

This may be more true of men than women. As part of their socialisation, men often come to associate worthwhile sex with intercourse leading to orgasm. One reason, therefore, why men may find it difficult to alter their sexual behaviour in the light of AIDS is that they do not regard safe sex as erotic. Another possible reason is that such changes would represent a threat to their identity and self-esteem. In our society sexual intercourse for men is often a way of achieving status and power over others, and is inextricably linked with being 'masculine'.

There are other reasons why AIDS may be more challenging to male sexuality than to female. With the onset of AIDS many men are experiencing what women have always experienced: an association between sex and danger. Fear of disease is only part of the dangers associated for women with sexuality. Alongside the possibility of sexual pleasure, fear of sexuality is traditionally instilled in women. Fear of being raped. Fear of becoming pregnant. Fear of being humiliated and hurt.

The association of death and desire is also nothing new for women. The physical harm done to victims of sexual violence reminds us of the fatal consequences sex can have for women. The threat of male violence is, however, not the only way in which sex for women has been linked with the possibility of death. Earlier this century it was not uncommon for women to die in childbirth. A woman's fear of sexuality, in this sense, was related to the prospect of repeated pregnancy.

The idea that there is a consequence to sexual behaviour has also resurfaced with AIDS. Men have been forced to consider risk, and to take responsibility for their actions. Again, this is something women have long had to deal with, whether in terms of the risk of pregnancy or of loss of reputation.

The challenge of AIDS is to create new meanings of sexuality that are not based on heterosexual intercourse or on men having more control over sexuality than women. Far from being a restrictive influence, we could see this as liberating for women, in terms of their relationships with men. However, the fear with AIDS is that it may lead to new forms of social control. Right-wing moralists are using AIDS as an argument for policies which would reverse the trends which are seen to have attacked marriage and the family. In this sense, AIDS is yet another example of the way in which the state, medicine and men regulate women's lives through their control over sexuality and reproduction.

Afterword

Writing about AIDS at the present time is rather like looking into a kaleidoscope; the picture keeps changing.

Towards the end of 1986 the British government, prompted by fears of AIDS spreading to the (hetero-sexual) population at large, launched a £20 million information campaign to combat AIDS. The campaign, entitled 'AIDS: Don't Die of Ignorance', included advertisements on billboards and radio, as well as in newspapers and magazines. In the New Year commercials about AIDS reached our television and cinema screens and, as I write, leaflets advising people how to avoid infection with HIV are on their way to 23 million homes.

It is a start. For many, however, the feeling is one of too little, too late. Spending £20 million on an advertising campaign may seem like a lot of money, but it is only a drop in the ocean in terms of what is needed.

Advertising campaigns are bound to lead to more people wanting to take the HIV antibody test. Yet the government has launched its public information campaign without providing extra funding to enable STD clinics to cope with the expected increased demand for testing and counselling. Nor has the government offered further funding for voluntary organisations like the Terrence Higgins Trust which, until recently, have provided much of the public information about AIDS and which continue to play a major role in offering help and advice.

Money is urgently needed elsewhere. We need a comprehensive long-term plan to develop health and social services to care for and support people with AIDS and those looking after them. We also need a massive research programme, not only to develop a cure and a vaccine, but also to study how people might be encouraged to change their sexual attitudes and behaviours, as well as their drug practices, in the light of AIDS.

What is already clear is that the government will have to do much more than distribute a free leaflet about AIDS and fund advertisements within the media to ensure that people understand about AIDS. We need a variety of campaigns directed at different groups, in language that is easy to understand, relevant to those it is aimed at and, most importantly, explicit. (It's no good having television advertisements telling people to protect themselves otherwise they might die from AIDS and never once mentioning the word condom.) Young people in particular need to be given information that is both understandable and relevant to them through the media and in schools. In addition, many parents are concerned about the risks their children face through sex or drug-use and feel they should talk to them about this. They may need advice about what, and how, to tell their children about AIDS.

Unfortunately for many women, both young and old, the facts will not be enough. Knowing about how to prevent HIV infection is not the same as feeling capable of putting that knowledge into practice. How many girls, for instance, are going to suggest, never mind insist, that their male partner wears a condom? Sex education should not just be about providing information. What is also needed are ways to help women to feel more assertive and say what they expect and want from sex.

Equally, if many men had a different attitude to sex women would not have to ask their male partners to use condoms. What is also required, therefore, are ways to encourage men to consider the risks of sex and not leave the responsibility for the safety of sex up to women. This will not be easy. Using a condom will have to be 'sold' to men through public advertising on TV and radio, in cinemas and in newspapers and magazines.

A major obstacle to this is the International Broadcasting Authority's ban on advertising condoms. Though it would undoubtedly be a major step forward if the IBA lifted its ban, it is not enough to tell people they ought to use condoms. Also needed are ways to help people to make changes in their sexual, or drug, practices. Condoms should be free and more easily available through chemists, doctor's surgeries, family planning and STD clinics, supermarkets and public toilets. It has also been suggested that they should be freely available in schools.

Similarly, free needles and syringes should be made available to drug users to stop them re-using infected ones. In some parts of the country schemes to provide drug users with free needles have already been set up. Those who inject drugs are given a new sterile injection kit free of charge when they hand in their old needles.

Developments occur quickly in discussions surrounding AIDS. Almost every day there is a new issue to consider. Until now AIDS in women has not received much attention. This is partly because, to date, it has been mainly men who have developed the disease (in the West). But this may not be the only reason. In the US, where over 2,000 women already have AIDS, funds to research women and AIDS have been virtually non-existent.

Apart from research, support groups for women are also needed. At present most such groups are for men. There is also a need for information services, including telephone helplines, specifically aimed at women. The Terrence Higgins Trust's leaflet 'Women and AIDS' is a welcome start. My concern however is that, as in other areas, women's needs will not be considered funding priorities. As more women become ill as a result of being infected with HIV, we must do everything we can to make sure that this does not happen and that women get the advice and the help they need.

Sheffield, January 1987

Note on sources

Very little has so far been written about women and AIDS. In researching this book I have therefore often had to make use of material which is not directly concerned with how the disease affects women. Books which are helpful in providing information on AIDS include the following.

AIDS: A Guide to Survival, Peter Tatchell, Gay Men's Press, 1986.

AIDS and the Blood, P. Jones, Haemophilia Society, 1985.

AIDS and the New Puritanism, Dennis Altman, Pluto Press, 1986.

AIDS Concerns You: What Every Man and Woman Should Know About AIDS, Jonathan Weber and Annabel Ferriman, Pagoda, 1986.

AIDS: Questions and Answers, V. G. Daniels, Cambridge Medical Books, 1986.

AIDS: The Deadly Epidemic, Graham Hancock and Enver Carim, Gollancz, 1986.

AIDS: The Story of a Disease, John Green and David Miller, Grafton, 1986.

The Management of AIDS Patients, ed. David Miller, Jonathan Weber and John Green, Macmillan, 1986.

Sex and Germs: The Politics of AIDS, Cindy Patton, South End Press, 1985.

The Truth About AIDS, Ann G. Fettner and William A. Check, Holt, Rinehart & Winston, 1984, reprinted 1985.

Understanding AIDS, Victor Gong, Cambridge University Press, 1985.

In writing this book, the following journals were an important source of information: *Annals of International Medicine*, *New England Journal of Medicine*, *American Journal of Medicine*, *British*

Medical Journal, Nature, Science, Journal of the American Medical Association, Cancer Research, British Journal of Obstetrics and Gynaecology, Community Care, Morbidity and Mortality Weekly Report, and *Communicable Disease Report.*

Reference was also made to material published by the Health Education Council, the Terrence Higgins Trust, the Haemophilia Society and various AIDS organisations both in the United Kingdom and the United States.

World and United States figures were obtained from the World Health Organisation (Paris) and the Centers for Disease Control (Atlanta, Georgia).

Sources for British figures included the DHSS, the Communicable Diseases Surveillance Centre, the Haemophilia Society, and the Home Office.

Resources list

Useful addresses

The Terrence Higgins Trust
BM/AIDS, London WC1N 3XX.
Telephone Helpline **01 833 2971.**
Monday to Friday 7p.m.-10p.m.; Saturday and Sunday 3p.m.-10p.m.

Offers help and counselling to people with HIV or AIDS, and their friends and relatives. Also provides an information service for those who are worried about AIDS. Has a drug group.

The Haemophilia Society
123 Westminster Bridge Road, London SE1 7HR.
Telephone **01 928 2020.**

Offers information and advice for people with haemophilia, their partners, friends and relatives.

Health Education Council
78 New Oxford Street, London WC1A 1AH.
Telephone **01 631 0930.**

Produces health education booklets on AIDS.

A free national telephone information and advice service on AIDS is available. The number is **0800 555777.** The taped message includes further numbers to call for information on a 24-hour basis.

Further information on AIDS can be obtained by using the *Healthline Telephone Service*. This is a 24-hour service providing recorded information on a number of AIDS-related issues. Telephone **01 981 2717** or **01 980 7222**. If you phone from outside London use the number **0345 581151** and you will be charged at local rates.

Women's Reproductive Rights Information Centre
52-54 Featherstone Street, London EC14 8RT.
Telephone **01 251 6332**.

Provides general information on women and AIDS.

SCODA (Standing Conference on Drug Abuse)
1-4 Hatton Place, London EC1N 8ND.
Telephone **01 430 2341**.

Has a full list of local services for drug users throughout the country. (During the times SCODA is not operating the Samaritans may be able to provide similar information by consulting the SCODA directory.) As some drug agencies may not know a great deal about AIDS, it may also be helpful to ring the Terrence Higgins Trust Drug Group.

London Lesbian and Gay Switchboard
BM Switchboard, London WC1N 3XX.
Telephone **01 837 7324** (24-hour service).

A telephone advisory and counselling service run by lesbians and gay men. Can answer general queries about AIDS and put you in touch with AIDS organisations and STD clinics.

STD clinics

STD clinics offer general advice about AIDS and can give you the HIV antibody test. They can also provide counselling for people who have AIDS or are antibody positive, and for their relatives and friends. You can refer yourself to an STD clinic. You don't need a letter from your doctor.

Most clinics are listed in the phone book under Sexually Transmitted Disease or Venereal Disease. Alternatively phone the local hospital, Family Planning Association or the British Pregnancy Advisory Service for the number. The FPA and the BPAS may also be able to provide useful information.

Regional AIDS groups

ENGLAND

Birmingham: AIDS line West Midlands
'Hazeliegh', 79 Stanmore Road, Edgbaston, Birmingham B16 9SU.
Telephone **021 622 1511.**
Tuesday and Thursday 7.30p.m.-10p.m. (answerphone at other times).

Bristol: Aled Richards Trust
1 Mark Lane, Bristol BS1 4XR.
Telephone **0272 273436.**
Thursday 7p.m.-9p.m. (answerphone at other times).

Leeds: AIDS Helpline
c/o Rockshots 2, 64-68 Call Lane, Leeds 2.
Telephone **0532 441661.**
Tuesday 7p.m.-9p.m.

Leeds: AIDS Advice
P.O. Box HP7, Leeds LS6 1PD.
Telephone **0532 444209.**
Monday and Thursday 7p.m.-9p.m. (recorded message at other times).

Liverpool: Merseyside AIDS Support Group
63 Shamrock Road, Birkenhead, L41 OEG.
Telephone **051 708 0234.**
Wednesday 7p.m.-10p.m.
or **051 246 8089** (recorded message giving details of clinics, AIDS support, etc.).

Manchester
P.O. Box 201, Manchester M60 1PU.
Telephone **061 228 1617**.
Monday to Friday 7p.m.-10p.m. (answerphone at other times).

Newcastle: AIDS North
Box NE 99 1BD, Newcastle-on-Tyne.
Telephone **091 232 2855.**

Oxford: OXAIDS
Freepost, Nether Westcote, OX7 6BR.
Telephone **0865 246036.**
Monday to Friday 10a.m.-12 noon, 1p.m.-5p.m.

WALES

Welsh AIDS Campaign Telephone **0222 464121.**

Gwent
Telephone (Caerlean) **0633 422 532.**
Tuesday 2p.m.-8p.m.
Telephone (Newport) **0633 841 901.**
Monday to Friday 8.30a.m.-4.30p.m.

SCOTLAND

Edinburgh and Glasgow: Scottish AIDS Monitor
P.O. Box 160, Edinburgh EH1 3UU.
Telephone (Edinburgh) **031 558 1167.**
Monday, Tuesday, Thursday and Friday 7.30p.m.-10p.m.

Telephone (Glasgow) **041 221 7467.**
Tuesday 7p.m.-10p.m.

NORTHERN IRELAND

Belfast: AIDS Belfast
c/o Cara Friend, P.O. Box 44, Belfast BT1 1SH.
Telephone **0232 226117.**
Friday 7.30p.m.-10.30p.m.

UNITED STATES

San Francisco: Women's AIDS Network
c/o San Francisco AIDS Foundation, 333 Valencia Street,
Fourth Floor, San Francisco, California 94103.

New York: Gay Men's Health Crisis
Box 274, 132 West 24th Street, New York, New York 10011.

AUSTRALIA

Sydney: AIDS Council of New South Wales (ACON)
P.O. Box 350, Darlinghurst, NSW 2010.
Telephone **(02) 332 4411** 10a.m.-6p.m.
Monday to Friday.
AIDS Hotline **(02) 332 4000.**

Melbourne: Victorian AIDS Council (VAC)
61-63 Rupert Street, Collingwood, Melbourne, NSW.
Postal address P.O. Box 174, Richmond, NSW 3121.
Telephone **(03) 417 1759.**

AIDS Line **(03) 419 3166** 7p.m.-10p.m.

Glossary

AIDS An abbreviation for Acquired Immune Deficiency Syndrome. It is a disease caused by a virus known as HIV, in which the body's immune system is seriously damaged. As a result people who have AIDS are susceptible to some rare cancers and often fatal infections.

AID Artificial Insemination by Donor. This is a simple procedure, by which sperm from a donor is placed in a woman's vagina using a syringe.

Anal intercourse (buggery; sodomy; rectal sex; arse-fucking) Sex where a man puts his penis into another person's rectum.

Antibodies Chemical substances developed by the immune system to fight infectious agents found in the body.

Antibody positive This is a blood test result showing that the person has been infected with HIV at some time. It does *not* mean a person has AIDS.

ARC Stands for AIDS-related complex. This refers to a group of people who have some symptoms of AIDS but who do not have any of the opportunistic infections and cancers associated with the disease. A significant proportion of people with ARC go on to develop AIDS.

Bisexual A woman or man who desires sexual relationships with both sexes.

Caesarean birth A method of childbirth in which a surgical incision is made through the abdominal wall and uterus.

Cervix The neck of the uterus or womb.

Clitoris ('clit') A small, complex organ located where the inside lips of the vagina meet. It plays an important role in women's orgasm.

Clitoridectomy The surgical removal of the clitoris and the inner and sometimes outer lips of the vagina.

Condom (sheath; rubber; johnny) A thin rubber sheath worn over a man's penis to reduce the risk of pregnancy, venereal disease, or infection with HIV.

Cunnilingus (oral sex; licking; sucking) When a person uses their tongue or mouth to stimulate a woman's genitals.

Ejaculation Discharge of semen (cum) from a man's penis.

Factor 8 An ingredient in the blood which is needed for the blood to clot normally.

Faeces Waste products; excrement; shit. 'Scat' is a slang term for sexual activities that involve faeces.

Fellatio (cock-sucking; blow job; giving head; oral sex) When a person uses their tongue or mouth to stimulate a man's penis.

Fisting (fist-fucking; hand-balling) This is where someone inserts their entire hand into another person's vagina or rectum.

French kiss A kiss that includes tongue contact and exchange of saliva (spit).

Gay A woman/man who finds other women/men sexually attractive and defines themselves as such (see also *Homosexual; Lesbian*).

Genitalia The external sex organs. In women this area is called the vulva and includes the inner and outer lips (labia) of the vagina, and the clitoris. In men this term refers to the penis, the scrotum and testicles (balls).

Gonorrhoea A sexually transmitted disease caused by bacteria.

Haemophilia A rare disease of the blood which mainly affects men. People with haemophilia need treatment to help their blood to clot (see also *Factor 8*).

Hand-to-genital sex (e.g. mutual masturbation; to wank someone off; hand job; finger-fucking) Where a person uses their hand or fingers to stimulate their partner's genitals.

Herpes A viral infection that produces painful blisters in the genital area.

Heterosexual ('straight') A term used to describe sexual relationships between women and men.

HIV Stands for human immunodeficiency virus. This is the name researchers have agreed upon for the virus which causes AIDS (see also *HTLV-3; LAV*).

HIV antibody test This is a blood test which shows whether or not a person has antibodies to the virus which causes AIDS. The test indicates only whether a person has at some time been infected with HIV. It cannot determine if a person has AIDS or will develop AIDS in future.

Homosexual (gay) Used to describe sex between two men and, to a lesser extent, two women. Also used to describe a *person* as homosexual or gay (see also *Gay; Lesbian*).

HTLV-3 or *Human T-cell Lymphotropic Virus Type-3.* This is the name American researchers first gave to the virus which causes AIDS.

Infibulation A form of clitoridectomy where the two sides of the vulva are sewn up after the clitoris has been removed.

Injecting drug user A person who injects drugs.

Intercourse (fucking; penetration; having sex) When a man puts his penis into a woman's vagina this is called vaginal intercourse. When he puts it into a person's rectum (back passage) this is called anal intercourse.

IUD Stands for intra-uterine device. This is a small plastic shape which can be inserted into a woman's womb to prevent pregnancy.

IV An abbreviation for intravenous. It is often used to describe drug users who inject drugs directly into their veins.

KS An abbreviation for Kaposi's sarcoma, a rare form of skin cancer which people with AIDS often get.

KY The brand name for a water-based lubricant for sex.

LAV Lymphadenopathy associated virus, the name French researchers first gave to the virus causing AIDS.

Lesbian (dyke; lezzie; gay) A woman who finds other women sexually attractive and defines herself as such.

Menstrual blood Blood that is shed from a woman's uterus during her period.

Monogamous Having sex with only one person.

Nonoxynol-9 A chemical agent in some spermicides and lubricants, which may reduce the risk of infection with HIV.

Opportunistic infections These are infections which take advantage of the opportunity offered by the body's weakened immune system to enter and cause illness.

Oral sex (see *Cunnilingus; Fellatio*).

Oral-anal sex (analingus; rimming) Where a person uses their mouth or tongue to stimulate another person's anus (arsehole; bumhole).

PCP An abbreviation of pneumocystis carinii pneumonia. This is a common illness in people with AIDS.

Penis (cock; dick; willie; prick; shaft) The male sex organ also used for urination (peeing).

PGL Stands for persistent generalised lymphadenopathy. This refers to a group of people who have persistently enlarged lymph glands, but who do not have any other symptoms of HIV infection. A proportion of people with PGL go on to develop AIDS.

PWA An abbreviation for people with AIDS.

Rectum (back passage) This is the lower part of the bowel, ending in the anus (arsehole; bumhole).

Semen (cum) Fluid ejaculated from a man's penis.

Sero-positive A person who has antibodies to HIV (see *Antibody positive*).

SI or *self-insemination* This is the term used when a woman carries out artificial insemination without the help of doctors or an official donor organisation.

Special clinic (see *STD clinic*).

Spermicide A chemical substance that kills sperm.

STDs (see also *VD*) An abbreviation for sexually transmitted diseases.

STD clinic (VD clinic; genito-urinary clinic) A clinic which specialises in dealing with sexually transmitted diseases.

T cells A group of white blood cells that protect the body against foreign agents, but which may be rendered ineffective by HIV.

Urine (wee; piss; pee).

Vagina (cunt) This is the organ in women leading from the vulva to the uterus or womb.

Vaginal intercourse (fucking; screwing; penetration; having sex; copulation; coitus) Sex where a man puts his penis into a woman's vagina.

VD Abbreviation for venereal disease. Any of a range of diseases that may be transmitted through sexual intercourse.

Vulva External sex organs in women; includes the outer and inner lips of the vagina and the clitoris.

Watersports A slang term for sexual activities that involve urine.

Works A term used by drug users to refer to equipment used for mixing or injecting drugs.

Index

Abortion, 50–1, 122, 128
Africa, 13, 17, 32, 33, 37, 40–4,
    53; incidence of AIDS in, 1,
    8–9, 11, 18, 40–1, 43; origin
    of AIDS in, 8–10; *see also*
    Racism; Third World
    Women; Transmission of
    HIV
AIDS (Acquired Immune
    Deficiency Syndrome), 3–6,
    142; cause of, 3, 6–8, 28, 31,
    49; discrimination, 27–8,
    85–9, 93, 108, 111, 114,
    118–19, 121, 125–8; funding,
    114, 115, 116, 117, 119, 120,
    123, 124; incidence of, 5, 10,
    11, 17–18, 25, 26, 27, 32, 61;
    incubation period, 5, 6, 8,
    117; and the media, 1, 11,
    17, 36, 46, 55, 91, 93, 116,
    117, 118, 126; origins of,
    8–10; symptoms of, 19–20,
    84, 91; *see also* HIV; People
    with AIDS; Treatment;
    Transmission of HIV
AIDS-related complex (ARC),
    4, 90, 142
Anal intercourse, 13, 32, 35,
    41, 73–5, 142, 144
Antibody test, 4–5, 17, 24, 25,
    29, 33, 46, 48, 53, 54, 60,
    122, 142; confidentiality,
    109, 111, 127; counselling
    for, 29, 50–1, 122, 125–6,
    128; negative test result, 5,
    47, 50–1, 125–6, 128; positive
    test result, 5, 47, 48, 50–1,
    85, 120, 122, 125–6, 128; the
    use of the test, 46, 47, 125–8;
    see also Artificial
    insemination; Blood
    donation; HIV
Artificial insemination, 18, 30,
    51–4, 55, 58, 59–61, 142;
    choosing a donor, 53–4; and
    lesbians, 51–2, 55, 58, 59–61;
    screening of donors, 53–4,
    59, 125, 128; self insemin-
    ation, 52, 53, 145;
    transmission of HIV virus
    by, 18, 30, 52–4
AWARE (Association for
    Women's Aids Research and
    Education), 24

Bereavement, 104; of lesbians,
    66–7
Bisexuality, 1, 15, 16, 17, 24,
    25, 33, 34, 37, 53, 57, 122,
    142

Blood and blood products, 16, 45–7, 110; transmission through, 1, 16, 18, 25, 36–41, 45–7, 110–11; *see also* Haemophilia

Blood donation, 41, 46, 47, 84, 125; by lesbians, 56–7; screening of donors, 17, 43, 46, 47, 59, 110, 125, 128

Breast feeding, transmission of HIV by, 14, 49–50, 84, 109, 112

Children with AIDS, 36, 43, 109–13, 121; incidence of, 43, 49, 109; precautions, 112 (*see also* Women caring for PWAs); school attendance, 111–12, 121; symptoms of, 110; transmission of HIV, 14, 43, 49–50, 59, 60, 84, 96, 110 (*see also* Pregnancy)

Condoms, 38, 68, 72, 74–5, 76–7, 79, 142

Contraception, 50, 77, 122

Drug use (injecting), 1, 18, 24, 25, 26–30, 36, 53, 58, 59, 93, 116, 118, 119, 138, 144; incidence of AIDS, 25, 26, 27, 28, 35, 36, 47; safer drug-use, 27, 28–9, 30, 126; sexual partners of injecting drug-users, 1, 18, 24, 27, 30, 32–3; transmission through shared needles, 26, 29, 30, 41, 44, 59, 65, 84

Education programmes, 29, 43–4, 50, 115–19, 126

Fisting, 64–5, 75, 76, 143

Gay men, 15, 16, 24, 28, 33, 82, 101, 108, 114, 116, 122, 125, 138, 143; as blood donors, 57; incidence of AIDS in, 1–2, 57, 59; scapegoating of, 9, 36–7, 93; as sperm donors, 53–4, 59; *see also* Homophobia; Lesbians

Haemophilia, 1, 18, 36, 53, 110, 111, 137, 143; children with, 110–11; incidence of AIDS, 16, 18; factor 8, 16, 33, 34, 110, 143; female partners of haemophiliacs, 16, 18, 24, 33, 34, 83

Haitians, 1, 44–5; incidence of AIDS, 44–5; origins of AIDS, 8, 45; transmission in, 24, 33, 44–5

Health-care workers, 12–13, 27, 106–9, 118; and AIDS discrimination, 27–8, 108, 118, 121; issues of confidentiality, 109, 111, 127; training, 108, 119, 120; risk of infection in, 12–13, 27–8, 106–7; risk reduction, 107

Heterosexual transmission, 13, 14, 15, 16, 18, 30–5, 41, 42, 43

HIV (human immuno-deficiency virus), 3, 4–8, 10–18, 20, 21, 23, 26, 36, 44, 49, 51, 59, 60; blood test for, 4–5, 142 (*see also* Antibody test); and brain damage, 5, 8, 48; as a cause of AIDS, 3, 6–8; symptoms of infection with, 19–20, 84, 91; vaccination against, 23, 115; *see also* Transmission of HIV

Homophobia, 2, 28, 67, 118, 126, 129

Hospice facilities, 120
Human T-cell Lymphotropic
  Virus-3 (HTLV-3), 3, 143

Immune system, 3, 5, 6, 7, 21,
  28, 42, 48, 49, 142, 144

Kaposi's sarcoma, 4, 19, 22,
  110, 144
Kissing, 32, 62, 63, 79–80, 143

Lesbians, 14, 55–67, 126, 138,
  144; with AIDS, 55, 57, 58,
  61, 65, 66–7; in AIDS
  organisations, 55, 56–7, 138;
  and artificial insemination,
  51–2, 55, 58, 59–61; and
  bisexual women, 34, 57;
  blood donations by, 56–7;
  and increased anti-gay
  feeling, 9, 55, 56, 126 (*see
  also* Homophobia); who
  inject drugs, 58, 59, 65;
  lesbian mothers, 52, 56, 59;
  safer-sex guidelines for,
  61–5; woman-to-woman
  transmission, 14, 34, 58,
  60–1
Lymphadenopathy associated
  virus (LAV), 3, 144
Lubricants, 72, 74, 77, 144

Masturbation, 63, 64, 80,
  143
Monogamy, 14, 15, 71, 144
Moral majority, 10

Nonoxynol-9, 74, 75, 77, 144

Opportunistic infections, 3,
  110, 142, 144
Oral sex, 32, 42, 62, 64, 78–9,
  144; cunnilingus, 32, 64, 78,
  79, 143; fellatio, 32, 78, 79,
  143; oral-anal sex, 32, 42, 64,

75, 78, 144 (*see also*
  Rimming)

People with AIDS (PWA), 103,
  144; discrimination against,
  86, 93, 108, 111, 114, 118,
  121, 123, 125–8; housing of,
  123–4, 126; isolation of,
  86–8; reactions to diagnosis,
  82–3, 92–3, 120; *see also*
  Women with AIDS
Persistent generalised
  lymphadenopathy (PGL), 4,
  90, 144
Pneumocystis carinii
  pneumonia (PCP), 3, 21–2,
  42, 110, 144
Policy issues, 111–13, 114–28;
  AIDS discrimination, 86,
  111, 114, 118, 121, 123,
  125–8; AIDS funding, 114,
  115, 116, 117, 119, 120, 123,
  124: community care for
  PWA, 105–6, 120, 121;
  education, 115–19, 126;
  health and social services,
  115, 119–23, 126; housing,
  123–4, 126; concerning
  children with AIDS, 111–13,
  121; the use of the HIV
  antibody test, 46, 47, 125–8
Pregnancy, 14, 47–51, 77, 81,
  82, 84, 96, 109, 110;
  transmission during, 14,
  48–50, 77, 96, 109, 110; *see
  also* Abortion; Contraception
Promiscuity, 10, 14, 15, 42, 129
Prostitutes, 10, 15, 27, 34,
  35–9, 43, 119, 125, 129;
  blaming AIDS on, 10, 35, 36,
  37, 38, 43, 93; registration
  of, 38; studies of HIV
  infection in, 35–6, 37, 43

Quarantine, 126

Racism, 2, 9, 40, 45
Rape, 39–40, 129
Rimming, 64, 75, 144; *see also*
  Oral sex
Risk-reduction, 13, 24, 71–5,
  78, 80, 84, 85, 107, 116, 125;
  see also Safer sex; Drug use

Safer sex, 13, 15, 27, 29, 32, 33,
  37, 60, 61–81, 85, 116, 117,
  126, 129; for heterosexual
  women, 27, 33, 68–81; for
  lesbians, 61–6
Sex toys, 62, 63, 64, 75, 78, 80,
  81
Sexuality, 15, 61–2, 129–30;
  changes in, 95–6, 129–30;
  construction of, 14, 36, 69;
  double standard, 14, 38;
  male sexuality, 38, 43, 69,
  129, 130; meaning to, 36, 43,
  68, 69, 129–31; sexual
  intercourse, 69, 72, 73, 74,
  75, 76–8, 129, 130, 144;
  women's experience, 68, 69,
  70, 130–1: lesbianism, 61–2;
  men's control over, 68, 69,
  71–3, 129, 130, 131; sexual
  difficulties, 61, 70, 95–6; *see
  also* Safer sex
STD clinics, 20, 104, 127, 138;
  145; *see also* Antibody test

T-cell, 6–7, 49, 145
Terrence Higgins Trust, 20, 88,
  116, 122, 137, 138
Third World Women, 11, 17;
  see also Africa
Transmission of HIV, 4, 5, 6,
  10–13, 15, 16, 26, 36, 44, 49,
  51, 59, 60, 112; in Africa, 9,
  18, 41, 43: blood
  transfusion, 13, 17, 41, 47;
  by insects, 9, 13, 41;
  heterosexual transmission,
  13–16, 18, 41, 42, 43; shared
  needles, 13, 16, 41, 43, 65;
  by artificial insemination,
  18, 30, 52–4; blood transfusion in, 17, 26, 45–7, 63:
  haemophilia, 16, 110–11;
  injecting drug use, 15, 16,
  18, 25, 26–30, 44, 63; in
  pregnancy, 14, 48–50, 109:
  breast feeding, 14, 49–50,
  109; risk to health workers,
  12–13, 27–8, 106–7; sexual,
  18, 30–5, 72–81: female–
  male, 13, 30, 31, 76, 78, 96;
  male–female, 13, 25, 30–4,
  39, 76, 77, 79; woman–
  woman, 14, 60–1, 62–6
Treatment, 10, 20–3, 92, 94–5,
  114, 119, 120; alternative,
  22–3, 94–5; antiviral drugs,
  20–1; immune-modulating
  drugs, 21

Vaccines, development of, 23,
  115
Vaginal intercourse, 39, 42, 51,
  73, 76–8, 145; transmission
  of HIV by, 13, 14, 42

Women with AIDS or who are
  antibody positive, 82;
  diagnosis, implications of,
  82–3, 92, 120: emotional, 82,
  83, 85, 87, 88–95; physical,
  82, 83, 84, 85, 87, 92; sexual,
  82, 89, 95–6; social, 82, 83,
  86, 87; discrimination
  against, 85, 86, 87, 119: in
  employment, 86, 89, 125,
  126; in health care, 86, 108,
  119, 126; in housing, 86, 126;
  in obtaining insurance, 86,
  125, 126, 127; incidence: in
  Africa, 11, 24, 35, 40–1, 43;
  in United Kingdom, 11–12,

17, 24, 27, 32, 47, 51; in
United States, 11, 24, 25–6,
27, 32, 35; precautions to
take, 84; pregnancy in, 14,
47–51, 71, 82, 84, 96, 109,
110; reactions of others to,
85, 86, 87, 89, 93, 120;
support groups for, 82, 86,
87–8, 122, 138; transmission
by, 60–1, 62–6, 83, 87
Women caring for PWA, 2, 12,
97–113, 118; with children
with AIDS, 109–13, 121, 122;
fear of infection in, 12–13,
27–8, 102, 104, 106–7, 110,
122; as health workers,
12–13, 27–8, 106–9; in the
home, 12, 97–101, 104–6,

120; policy issues, 105–6,
108, 109, 111, 112–13, 120–2;
precautions, 102, 104, 107,
112; support groups for,
101, 104, 120, 122
Women at risk, 2, 13, 71–81,
84; injecting drug users, 1,
18, 24, 25, 26–30, 35, 36, 47,
58–9, 118, 119; sexual
partners of bisexual or gay
men, 2, 15, 16, 24, 25, 32–4,
37, 53, 57, 71–5: of injecting
drug users, 1, 18, 24, 27, 30,
32–3; of haemophiliacs, 16,
18, 24, 33, 34, 83; *see also*
Lesbians; Prostitution; Rape;
Third World Women